MW00386816

EASY COOKBOOK FOR HEALTHY, WHOLESOME RECIPES

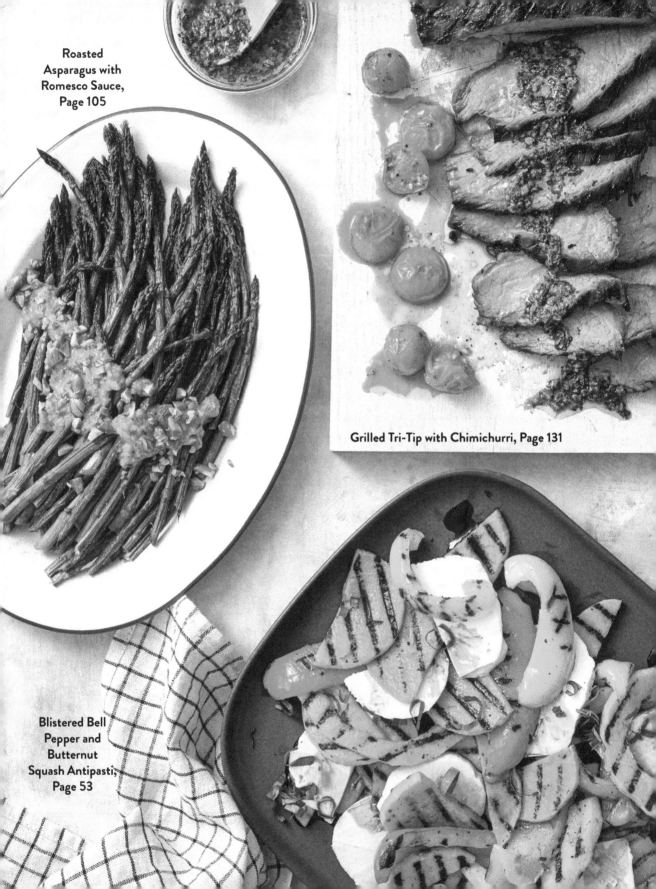

Roasted Asparagus with Romesco Sauce, Page 105

Grilled Tri-Tip with Chimichurri, Page 131

Blistered Bell Pepper and Butternut Squash Antipasti, Page 53

EASY COOKBOOK

— FOR —

HEALTHY, WHOLESOME RECIPES

Anja Lee Wittels

Photography by Kate Sears

ROCKRIDGE
PRESS

Copyright © 2021 by Rockridge Press, Emeryville, California

No part of this publication may be reproduced, stored in a retrieval system, or transmitted in any form or by any means, electronic, mechanical, photocopying, recording, scanning, or otherwise, except as permitted under Sections 107 or 108 of the 1976 United States Copyright Act, without the prior written permission of the Publisher. Requests to the Publisher for permission should be addressed to the Permissions Department, Rockridge Press, 6005 Shellmound Street, Suite 175, Emeryville, CA 94608.

Limit of Liability/Disclaimer of Warranty: The Publisher and the author make no representations or warranties with respect to the accuracy or completeness of the contents of this work and specifically disclaim all warranties, including without limitation warranties of fitness for a particular purpose. No warranty may be created or extended by sales or promotional materials. The advice and strategies contained herein may not be suitable for every situation. This work is sold with the understanding that the Publisher is not engaged in rendering medical, legal, or other professional advice or services. If professional assistance is required, the services of a competent professional person should be sought. Neither the Publisher nor the author shall be liable for damages arising herefrom. The fact that an individual, organization, or website is referred to in this work as a citation and/or potential source of further information does not mean that the author or the Publisher endorses the information the individual, organization, or website may provide or recommendations they/it may make. Further, readers should be aware that websites listed in this work may have changed or disappeared between when this work was written and when it is read.

For general information on our other products and services or to obtain technical support, please contact our Customer Care Department within the United States at (866) 744-2665, or outside the United States at (510) 253-0500.

Rockridge Press publishes its books in a variety of electronic and print formats. Some content that appears in print may not be available in electronic books, and vice versa.

TRADEMARKS: Rockridge Press and the Rockridge Press logo are trademarks or registered trademarks of Callisto Media Inc. and/or its affiliates, in the United States and other countries, and may not be used without written permission. All other trademarks are the property of their respective owners. Rockridge Press is not associated with any product or vendor mentioned in this book.

Interior and Cover Designer: Eric Pratt
Art Producer: Hannah Dickerson
Editor: Van Van Cleave
Photography © 2021 Kate Sears, food styling by Lori Powell
Illustrations © 2021 Claire McCracken

ISBN: Print 978-1-64876-625-1 | eBook 978-1-64876-124-9

R1

To my biggest cooking and
innovation inspirations—Mom, Dad, Kelsey,
Mason, Spencer, Mimi, Melanie & Sylvie

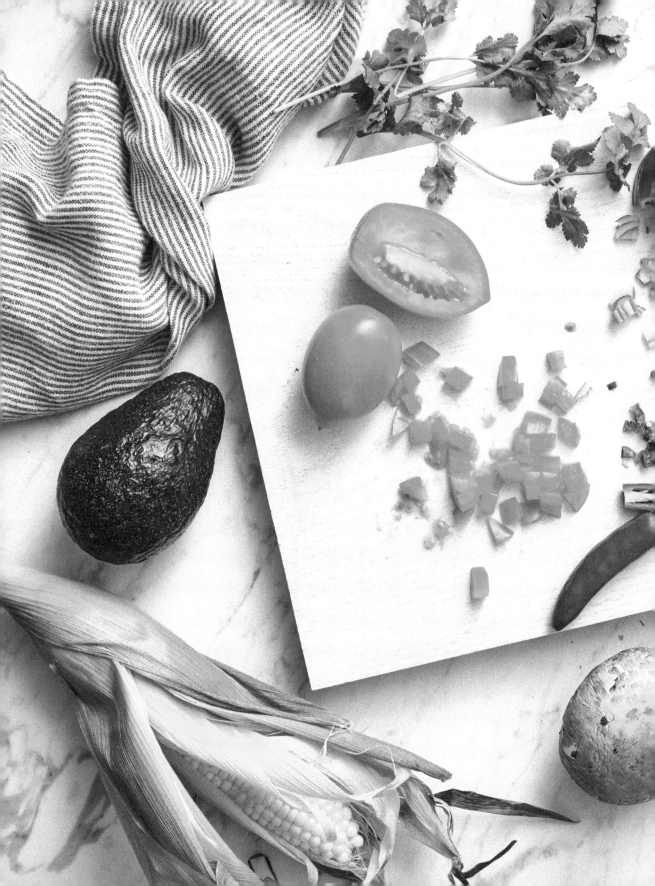

Contents

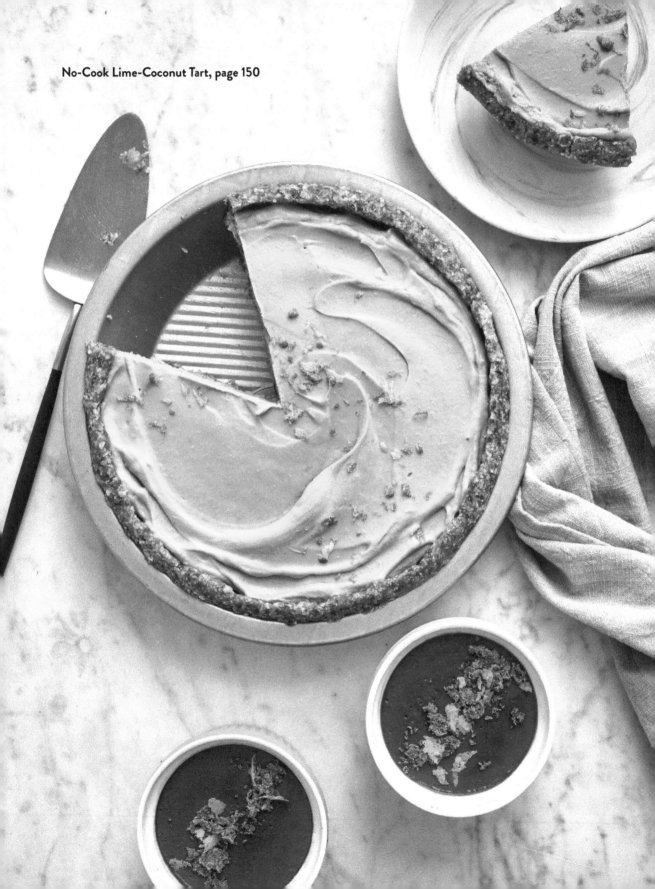

No-Cook Lime-Coconut Tart, page 150

Introduction

Welcome to the world of easy, healthy cooking! It's a snap to make many recipes more nutritious with just a few adjustments, even for the novice cook. You just need to understand the basics.

This book is the perfect introduction to learning everything you need to know to cook delicious, nourishing meals. The most important part of cooking is getting yourself into the kitchen. The next step is practicing the techniques for success that I outline in this book.

I treasure the memories of my first moments in the kitchen while cooking with my mom. One night, in my early double-digit years, she let me cook dinner for the family. I chose the recipe based on some beautiful photos in one of her cookbooks, then I shopped with her for the ingredients at the grocery store. Once back home, I mixed up a marinade, roasted a juicy steak, and made a chimichurri to drizzle on top. Believe it or not, the meal turned out well! This dinner was a magical moment, and it was then that I knew I loved cooking for others and myself.

Over the years, I have learned all sorts of tricks to cook healthier food that I am excited to share with you in this book. Whether roasting at the correct temperature to preserve a food's nutrients or avoiding harmful oils, I demonstrate all sorts of important techniques for stress-free, healthier cooking. Once these skills are learned, the rest of the recipes in this book, and many other books after, will be a piece of cake! Even in the simplest kitchen setup, this book will be a secret weapon for cooking delicious, satisfying, wholesome, and energizing food for you and your whole family!

1

BACK TO BASICS

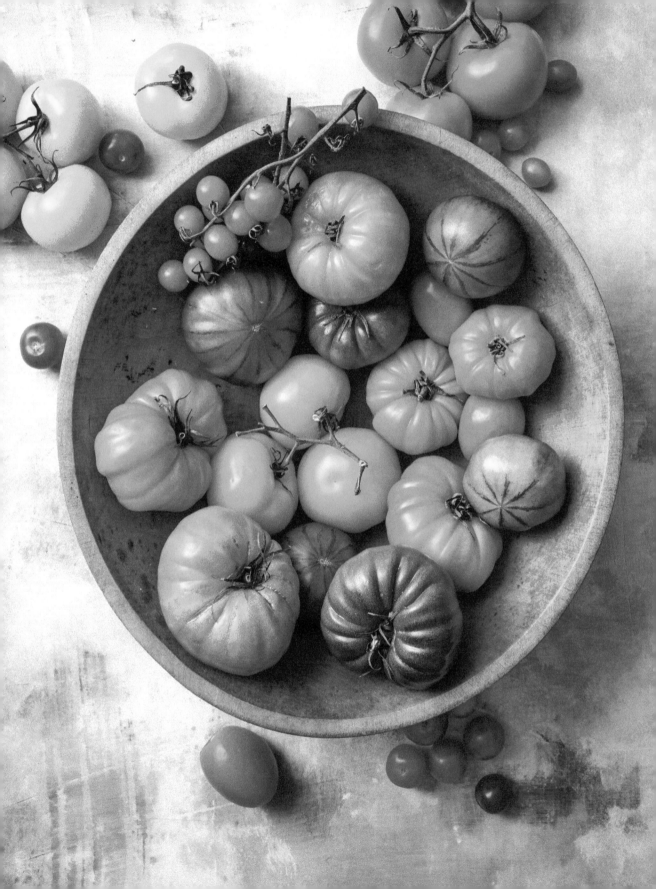

CHAPTER ONE

A FRESH START

- - - - -

Getting started can be the toughest part of cooking. In this chapter, we'll discuss how to begin—from using your senses and choosing kitchen equipment to how to grocery shop and what to stock in your pantry.

Wholesome at Its Simplest

There are countless benefits to cooking at home. There's the unbeatable satisfaction of having made something with your own hands that you and your loved ones can enjoy. This is especially true when you cook together, and this can be the perfect time of day to catch up with each other. We frequently save money when we grocery shop for ourselves, as it allows us to choose what to buy and where to buy it. More than anything, home-cooked meals are often healthier, since you know exactly what ingredients are going into the food. This includes adding nourishing olive oil instead of unhealthy canola oil, enhancing the flavor with mineral-rich sea salt instead of nutrient-stripped kosher salt, and adding anti-inflammatory spices such as turmeric and cinnamon. Many may consider cooking time consuming. But really, cooking for ourselves can be a time-saver when taking into account the amount of time spent waiting to order food and then the delivery time for it to arrive.

This book will help define the principles of healthy cooking and how such a task can be done in the comfort of your home, often with only about 20 minutes of active time involved. I take you through a few easy recipes to practice, beginning with a simple and scrumptious Southwest-Style Quinoa (page 25) that offers a meal rich in protein, fiber, and amino acids. Then, we'll make fiber-rich Black Beans with Garlic and Cumin (page 26) and heart-healthy Swiss Chard Tortillas (page 28). Later in this book, you will master some of my favorite recipes, which are easy and absolutely delicious, including Grilled Heirloom Tomatoes with Spicy Tahini Dressing (page 85), Grilled Tri-Tip with Chimichurri (page 131), and a MUST in my kitchen: Anja's Dark Chocolate–Berry Crumble (page 149)—because even healthy cooking includes a few treats.

Tips for Getting to Good

My hope is that you come to realize that cooking delicious, healthy food is not difficult. It simply requires a few fresh ingredients, a fairly well-stocked pantry, the right tools to cook with, and, of course, your eyes, ears, nose, and mouth. With that, here are seven general guidelines to follow to ensure healthy cooking is successful and stress-free.

1. **Trust your senses.** Recipes are wonderful road maps to a finished dish, but at the end of the day, senses and instincts will tell if something is off—or just needs a little tweaking.

2. **Be adventurous choosing vegetables.** When you cook with vegetables harvested during the proper season, they will be innately flavorful. Usually, a little salt and olive oil is enough to enhance their flavor.

3. **Shop with awareness.** When grocery shopping, make a conscious effort to read the labels, so you know where your food comes from and what's in it. If you are adhering to a gluten-free diet, always check ingredient packaging for gluten-free labeling (in order to ensure foods, especially oats, were processed in a completely gluten-free facility).

4. **Work with what's available.** Allow the ingredients you find at the grocery store or farmers' market to inspire what you cook. It's easy to become attached to a specific idea for a recipe, but if the ingredients are not available or not in season, it's likely the dish will not turn out as hoped.

5. **Cook simply.** Healthy food doesn't need to be complex, and often it is better if the ingredients maintain their flavor and composition. They can be delicious using simple cooking techniques.

6. **Taste.** Similar to trusting your senses, it is important to taste at every step of the process so that you understand the flavors you are using and ensure that you are not adding too little or too much of them. A recipe is a guide, not the rule book.

7. **Cook and eat together!** Our fast-paced lives don't always allow for sit-down meals. But it is important to prioritize those moments when we can share the pleasure of cooking and eating with friends and family.

Kitchen Essentials

Having the proper equipment in the kitchen makes all the difference. It's not necessary to have equipment in abundance. Instead, focus on fewer pieces, and make sure they are made well, versatile, and will last a long time. The following are must-haves in my kitchen:

3-quart saucepan: Use for boiling water, making sauces, and heating liquids.

8-quart stockpot: This is the perfect pot for making large quantities of stock or boiling pasta and potatoes.

10-inch cast-iron skillet: This is your go-to tool for dinner most nights—durable and versatile, super easy to clean, can be used on the stovetop and in the oven, nonstick, free of chemicals, and, when heated, retains its heat.

Baking sheets and dishes: Use for all roasting purposes. Cooking with the oven is fantastic—it is low maintenance.

Chef's knife: This multipurpose knife can be used for chopping, dicing, and mincing vegetables, meats, or anything that requires something larger than a paring knife. If there is one knife to invest in, it is this one. A sharp, high-quality knife is safer and easier to use.

Colander: This tool is useful when washing vegetables and fruits or straining pastas or other foods. A metal colander is best.

Cutting board: A *large board* will be essential for chopping onions, garlic, vegetables, meats, or anything that requires a good-size workspace; a *small board* for smaller fruits, vegetables, cheeses, and the like.

Measuring cups and spoons: Use for measuring precise amounts of ingredients.

Mixing bowls: Ideally stainless steel, ceramic, or glass, use these for mixing ingredients.

Rubber spatula: This tool is great for scraping out all the contents from the bowl or pan, decreasing waste.

Serrated knife and paring knife: These two knives will be helpers when the chef's knife just doesn't cut it (literally!). The teeth of the serrated knife—similar to a saw—are perfect for cutting things like bread and tomatoes that have a hard exterior and soft interior. A paring knife is ideal for cutting smaller items like fruits, vegetables, cheeses, or anything that requires a bit more detailed work.

Stainless-steel or ceramic sauté pan or skillet: These pans can be used for many purposes, such as sautéing, searing, and making sauces.

Tongs: Use these for mixing, flipping, transferring, and even serving.

Wooden spoons: Use these for all your mixing, stirring, and sautéing needs.

HOW POTS AND PANS STACK UP

The number of cookware options available can seem daunting, from nonstick to copper, aluminum, and stainless steel. These guidelines can help you make informed decisions.

Aluminum versus cast iron: Aluminum is lightweight and an excellent heat conductor; however, similar to copper, it can be reactive with acidic foods like tomatoes, citrus, and vinegar. This is why you'll sometimes find that food has picked up a slight metallic taste when cooked in aluminum. Though aluminum may not pose a health threat, cast iron is a better option. It is a great heat conductor, is super durable, and can be used on the stovetop, oven, and grill.

Copper versus stainless steel: Copper pots are beautiful and heat quickly and evenly. However, when acidic foods are made in uncoated cookware, the pots can release copper, which, in excess amounts, can lead to heavy metal poisoning. And when copper is coated, the coating often contains nickel. Stainless steel is a better option. It is scratch resistant and can be seasoned to make it nonstick. Look for food-grade stainless steel that doesn't contain any nickel.

Teflon versus ceramic: Teflon, also known as PTFE, is used as a nonstick coating for pans, making them convenient and easy to clean. If overheated, the coating can break down, releasing toxic particles and gases. A comparable option is ceramic, which is also nonstick and easy to clean. Ceramic cookware is regarded as safer than PTFE because its coating is apparently nontoxic, though the evidence remains inconclusive.

Healthier Shopping

Grocery shopping once a week is a great time-saver. Having meals, or at least ideas for meals, planned for the week becomes useful when it's 6 p.m. on Wednesday and you're feeling hungry and uninspired. Not to mention, your ingredients will be fresher than when bought in bulk weeks ahead. But if that's not feasible or your style, it's a plus to have pantry staples on hand that make it possible to whip up a healthy meal in no time. Think pastas, grains, and legumes, such as quinoa, polenta, rice, chickpeas, and black beans. These ingredients last for months and can be transformed into a variety of dishes. When navigating the grocery store, stick to the outer aisles, where you'll find most of the produce, meats, fish, and generally healthier options. Take a stroll through the grains and canned goods aisle, where you'll find much of what you'll need to round out your pantry.

Pantry Staples

Most good kitchens have a well-stocked pantry filled with these long-lasting essentials, providing the tools to create a diverse range of dishes. Once you have these ingredients stocked, you won't have to worry about what's on hand, lessening some of that stress of meal planning and preparation.

- Baking powder and baking soda
- Beans, dried or canned: black, cannellini, chickpeas, kidney
- Black pepper (preferably whole peppercorns and a grinder); once pepper is ground, it quickly begins to lose its flavor
- Cooking oils: extra-virgin olive and coconut
- Essential ground spices and dried herbs: basil, cardamom, cayenne, cinnamon, cloves, coriander, cumin, ginger, nutmeg, oregano, paprika, red pepper flakes, rosemary, thyme
- Farro and barley
- Flour: all-purpose, almond, buckwheat, gluten-free 1:1, spelt
- Garlic: dried and fresh

- Pastas: whole-wheat and other healthy alternatives, such as chickpea and edamame
- Quinoa
- Rice: black, brown, jasmine
- Salt (preferably fine sea salt)
- Sweeteners: honey, maple syrup, white cane or coconut sugar
- Tomatoes, canned: chopped, pureed, or both
- Vinegars: apple cider, balsamic, red wine, rice wine, sherry, white wine
- Vanilla extract

Fresh + Frozen Ingredients

A healthy diet should comprise primarily fresh ingredients, though there's plenty of evidence that frozen fruits and vegetables retain a high amount of nutrients, too. And, if having frozen produce in your freezer makes it easier to cook healthy, go for it. Some lean proteins and cheeses can also be frozen. Be sure to freeze any ingredients when they are at the ripeness or freshness you like because the cold temperatures will stop their ripening process. For safety and best flavor, be sure frozen ingredients are completely thawed before cooking with them.

- Cheese: feta, goat's milk, Gruyère, mozzarella, parmesan
- Eggs
- Flavor enhancers: garlic, lemon, lime, onion
- Fruit: apples, berries, peaches, pears
- Greens: arugula, butter lettuce, kale, red leaf lettuce, spinach, Swiss chard
- Hearty vegetables: bell peppers, broccolini, carrots, fingerling potatoes, squash, sweet potatoes
- Lean proteins: chicken, fish, lamb, shellfish, turkey
- Milk: cow's or nut
- Yogurt, plain: goat's milk and Greek

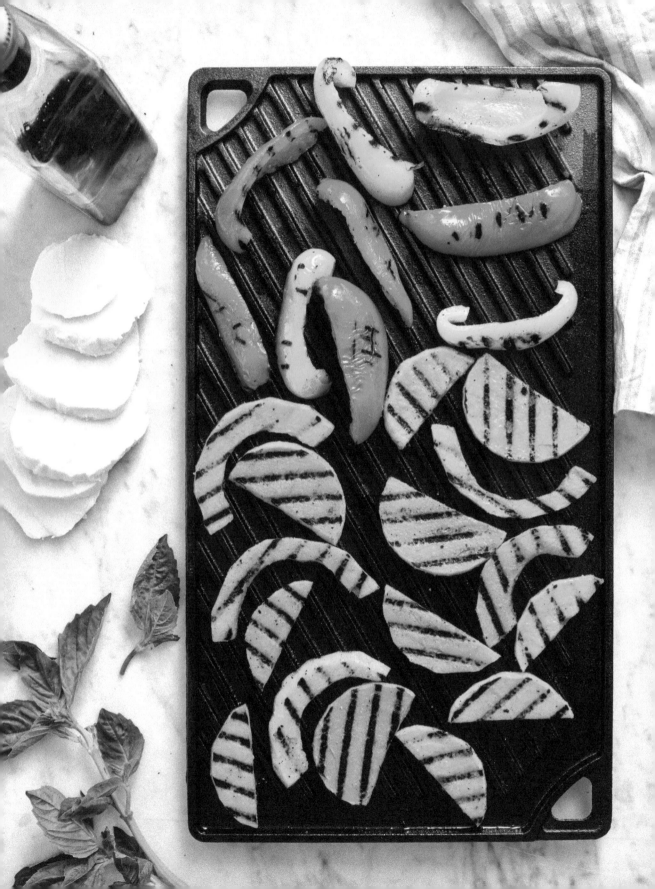

CHAPTER TWO

FEEL-GOOD COOKING

Food shouldn't just taste good; it should leave you feeling light, fresh, and full of energy. In this chapter, we'll move beyond just foods that are tasty and learn everything you need to maximize the benefits of your healthy culinary creations.

Designing Easy, Healthy Meals

As you strive to cook healthier, remember, every meal doesn't have to take up a significant portion of your day. By keeping to a few key themes, you can whip up a quick, healthy, hearty meal for yourself or many.

If it grows, it goes: Throw lots of veggies and fruit into the mix. My favorite trick is to pick a medley of veggies, chop them, throw in some SPOOG (salt, pepper, olive oil, and garlic powder; see recipe on page 18), and sauté them in a hot pan. It's easy to do, fills the kitchen with wonderful aromas, and guarantees you receive the fiber and nutrients your body needs every day.

Whole grains: Pasta, quinoa, and rice are great options for a quick fix and are tasty complements to the veggies you have cooking in the pan. Whole grains offer fiber, minerals, protein, and essential carbohydrates your body needs to stay strong. If you choose a grain, opt for the "whole" (less processed) option. Aim for ¼ cup dried grain portion per person (the grains expand while cooking).

Lean, mean protein: Meats can be done properly—and fast. When choosing the right meat for your meal, select leaner options, especially when it comes to ground red meats (shoot for 85 or 90 percent lean). You won't lose too much flavor, and you can add flavor with seasonings. Meat should not be the star of the show but rather a complement (a portion the size of your fist) to the healthy vegetables and grains on your plate.

Fat fattens: One of the best ways to fight off the fat is to keep it out of your food. Although there are some healthy fats, get creative with different ways to flavor or moisten foods. Squeeze on lemon juice, add yogurt, toss in a light olive oil. Don't just cover it in butter.

Saved by the seasoning: Adding spices and herbs can give your body the extra minerals and antioxidants it needs. Know that store-bought, premade seasonings usually contain preservatives and added sugars that are not good for your body. But, whether you're a salt and pepper purist or the proud owner of a 500-piece spice rack, the most important thing is to use the spices while they're fresh. And the trick to using seasonings while fresh is to figure out what you like. Remember to taste as you season. When in doubt, add more.

On the Safe Side

I can already smell the sweet aromas from your kitchen. So, now that you're inspired to start making healthier foods for yourself and your family, there are a few food safety items to know. I call it SICS, short for "Supermarket, In the Kitchen, Cleaning, and Storage." After all, when cooking healthier, the last thing you want to do is to make yourself or someone else sick. Here's what you need to know:

Supermarket

- Check products' expiration dates.
- Smell meat, cheese, and other foods to make sure the aroma is not funky (remember, trust your instincts!).
- Shop for perishables last so they don't spoil.
- Separate raw foods, i.e., the meats from the vegetables.

In the Kitchen

- Handle raw meat with care. Wash your hands after handling it, and don't mix it with other foods until cooked.
- Cook ground beef, lamb, pork, or veal until it's no longer pink, or until it reaches an internal temperature of at least 160°F. But if you like your meat on the rare side, feel free to leave it very pink.
- Cook chicken and other poultry until it's no longer pink, or until it reaches an internal temperature of at least 165°F.
- Cook eggs thoroughly so whites are firm. It is okay to leave the yolk runny (sunny-side up is great!). Scrambled eggs should not be runny.

Cleaning

- Make sure your hands are clean: simple but true!
- Scrub all fruits and veggies with plain water to remove any pesticides, dirt, or bacterial contamination.
- Clean all utensils and workspaces each time you use them (counters, cutting boards, etc.). These can easily contain bacteria.
- Use hot water and soap.
- Clean towels in hot water.

Storage

- Put leftovers in the refrigerator soon after you've finished with them.
- Store everything in a container with a tight-fitting lid.
- Eat leftovers within 3 to 4 days.
- If you freeze leftovers, eat them within 2 months.

HOW TO KNOW WHEN IT'S "DONE"

Different foods have different points of "doneness." Here, I offer general rules for recognizing doneness in certain grains and meats. This will be an easy point of reference when it comes to cooking these ingredients. I highly recommend investing in a meat thermometer.

FOOD	WHEN IT'S DONE
Beans	Softened but not mushy
Beef	Rare: 120°F to 130°F; medium-rare: 130°F to 135°F; medium-well: 145°F to 155°F
Beef, ground	Cook for 7 to 10 minutes over medium-high heat to minimum internal temperature of 160°F
Chicken	165°F; juices run clear
Fish	Firm to the touch; not translucent
Grains	All the water is absorbed; not hard but not too soft
Lamb	Medium-rare: 130°F to 135°F; medium: 135°F to 145°F; well: 160°F
Pasta	Al dente, with a bit of texture, but not too soft
Pork	Medium: 145°F to 150°F; well: 160°F
Rice	Not crunchy; not too soft
Sausage	160°F; no pink inside
Veal	Medium-rare: 130°F to 135°F; medium: 135°F to 145°F; well: 160°F

Simply Delicious

One trick I have found to make healthier cooking a habit is nailing flavor. Here are some ingredients and methods to keep in mind to ensure your food turns into something your body and taste buds crave just from that energized feeling after eating it.

Salt

There are many types of salts, and some are more flavorful than others. Unprocessed salt, such as sea salt or Himalayan salt, has crystals that are much saltier, meaning you need less of it to enhance your food. When working with these high-quality salts, add them closer to the end of cooking because salt brings out liquid in food and can interfere with the browning process when searing. Once the food is warm and cooked, it will absorb the salt nicely, and the salt will enhance the flavor. A little healthy salt in your diet is key to receiving the minerals your body needs to regulate fluid and muscle function. When using a processed table or kosher salt, your food will require more to taste good and overwhelm your body with sodium. Too much sodium causes your body to retain water and can lead to gaining unhealthy weight. So, choose a fine sea salt or other healthier, less processed salt.

Pepper

Pepper comes in many different forms. We typically use dried, ground forms. You will also find spicy cayenne pepper and red pepper flakes as flavoring options. Whole peppercorns, another option, are flavor enhancers that add a warming sensation to your food but don't necessarily make food spicy. Peppercorns come in different colors: black, green, pink, red, and white, with black being the most common. Each adds a different flavor to your food. Freshly ground peppercorns impart the most flavor. When using pepper, I find adding a little at the beginning of cooking enhances the pepper flavor as it touches the heat. If needed, add pepper at the end as well for a fresher, brighter pepper flavor.

Healthy Fats

Fats have a bad reputation. Some fats are considered "healthy" fats, including olive oil, whole milk, coconut, avocado, flaxseed, and nuts. All offer essential nutrients for your body that help protect your muscles and organs. Use them lightly, since they can cause weight gain. Fats also enhance dishes significantly, introducing new flavor to them and making them heartier and more satisfying. Olive oil, for instance, can add a Mediterranean-style soft flavor.

Fresh + Dried Herbs

Whether fresh or dried, herbs enhance foods significantly. I tend to use fresh basil, cilantro, dill, parsley, and thyme in many of my dishes though I lean toward oregano and tarragon in dried form. Once you test them both ways, you will learn your preference. Either way, you cannot go wrong adding herbs to every dish.

Spice Mixes

Spices are dried, and therefore a little goes a long way. If they are added to something that is cooked, their flavor is enhanced by the heat. Some spices are better added at the beginning of the cooking process, whereas others are better added at the end. This is because some spices, such as turmeric or cumin seed, need time to develop their flavor, whereas others are better fresh, like cinnamon.

Vinegars + Citrus Juice

One important step many cooks forget is to brighten the flavors of their food with an acid. When a dish feels like it is missing something, just a little bit of vinegar or citrus juice can bring it to life.

Dried Vegetables + Fruit

Dried vegetables and fruit are great for cooking with in winter, when fresh foods are not as plentiful. Dried fruits are also flavorful additions to salads, as well as sweet and savory cooked dishes. When dried, the flavor of fruit is concentrated. Therefore, when rehydrated, dried fruit infuses tons of flavor into dishes.

Marinades

To make a meat or vegetable stand out with flavor, make a marinade by mixing a combination of salt, pepper, herbs, spices, acid, and healthy fats. Then let the meat or vegetable sit in it for at least 1 hour before cooking. The marinade will seep into the ingredient and add tons of flavor.

Bastes

To maintain the moisture in a food that is cooking, generously baste with the juices and fats at the bottom of the pan. Use a spoon, scoop up the juices, and give the food a nice bath of flavor.

MINI RECIPE: SPOOG

This recipe is referenced many times within the book, so make sure to note this page! SPOOG is an easy way to add the perfect amount of healthy flavor to almost anything—meat or vegetable. It can be baked, sautéed, added after poaching, and even eaten raw in a salad dressing or sauce.

½ teaspoon sea salt (S)

¼ teaspoon freshly ground black pepper (P)

1 tablespoon extra-virgin olive oil (OO)

½ teaspoon garlic powder (G)

In a bowl, using a whisk or fork, mix together the salt, pepper, oil, and garlic powder. Store in a tightly sealed container at room temperature for months. The oil and salt act as preservatives; as long as no water gets into the container, there should not be room for growth of any bad bacteria.

About the Techniques + Recipes

I've chosen these recipes and techniques to demonstrate progressively how to cook delicious healthy foods easily and enjoyably. Starting with guidelines to make cooking successful and stress-free to stocking your kitchen with proper equipment and your pantry with key ingredients, from grocery shopping to planning meals and everything in between, this cookbook gives you the tools to cook healthy foods simply and help you lead an overall more balanced lifestyle.

The techniques and Try It! practice recipes in part 2 progress in stages, starting with basic healthy cooking methods for a solid skills foundation leading to recipes that bring it all together in part 3. Each recipe contains a description, yield, active time, allergy labels, ingredients, and, of course, directions. I even add tips to make a recipe step or working with an ingredient easier; include healthy swaps to make a dish vegan or vegetarian, gluten-free, lower carb, lower fat, or lower sodium; and include a few next-level techniques to consider if you feel adventurous.

Take your time, enjoy the ride, and taste as you go. Food and eating are about nourishing your body and enjoying it in good company. You have the freedom to taste as you cook and learn as you go, so don't be afraid to take a taste at every step to "make sure the food isn't poisonous" (as my mom would say), or better yet, make sure it is scrumptious!

ESSENTIAL
TECHNIQUES + RECIPES

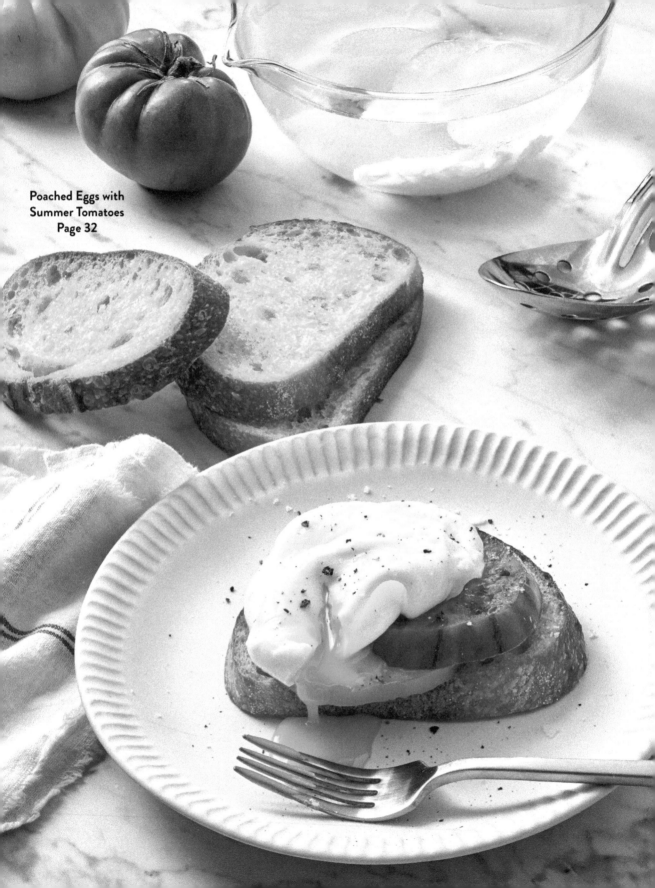

Poached Eggs with
Summer Tomatoes
Page 32

CHAPTER THREE

COOKING WITH WATER

In this chapter, you'll learn the basics of cooking with water—from boiling to blanching, steaming, and poaching. Cooking with water is versatile, simple, and healthy.

How to Boil Water

Cooking with water is incredibly simple. It also requires virtually no fat, leading to very clean and healthy eating. When sautéing, frying, grilling, or roasting, usually some fat is necessary, though it's not always a bad thing. If you want to avoid the use of fats, cooking with water is the way to go. When cooking with water, it is important to differentiate between a rolling boil and simmering. At a rolling boil, the water forms large, strong bubbles, and the temperature is 212°F. At a simmer, the water bubbles more slowly and steadily, and the temperature is below 212°F. When cooking pasta, bring the water to a rolling boil before adding the pasta, then stir it; otherwise the pasta will stick together.

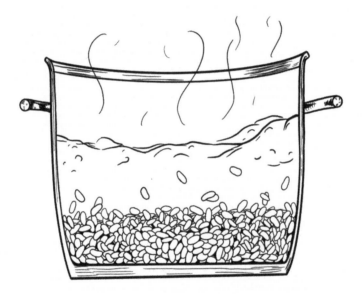

Boil

In most recipes that use boiling as the cooking method, you start by bringing the water to a rolling boil so it is incredibly hot and powerful. Then, after adding your ingredient, adjust the heat down to a simmer, so it cooks slowly and steadily, without too much water evaporating quickly. Ingredients that are great for cooking with this method are grains, beans, rice, pastas, potatoes, eggs, and meats—usually tougher cuts that need to be cooked for a long time, such as brisket.

Southwest-Style Quinoa

SERVES 3 OR 4 / ACTIVE TIME: 20 MINUTES

DAIRY-FREE, GLUTEN-FREE, NUT-FREE, VEGETARIAN

Quinoa, considered the "super grain of the future," dates back three to four thousand years, when the Incas believed it increased the stamina of their warriors. It is a complete protein containing all nine essential amino acids, which is better than what most meats provide. Enjoy this as a side with almost anything, including Lemon-Tarragon Salmon and Roasted Broccolini (page 124) as well as Turkey Meatballs with Warm Spinach Yogurt (page 143).

1 tablespoon extra-virgin olive oil

½ yellow onion, chopped

1 cup quinoa, rinsed

1 teaspoon sea salt

2 cups water

½ teaspoon ground cumin

½ teaspoon chili powder

½ teaspoon garlic powder

1. Preheat a small pot over medium heat.
2. When the pot is hot, pour in the oil, and add the onion. Sauté, stirring occasionally, for about 3 minutes, or until the onion starts to look translucent.
3. Stir in the quinoa, and add the salt. Immediately stir in the water.
4. Increase the heat to high.
5. As soon as the water comes to a boil (large bubbles form), reduce the heat to medium-low, and bring to a simmer. Cook for 15 minutes, or until the water has been absorbed into the quinoa. If not, cook for 1 to 2 minutes more, or until no water remains but the quinoa is not burning on the bottom of the pot.
6. Stir in the cumin, chili powder, and garlic powder. Remove from the heat. Cover the pot, and let sit for at least 10 minutes before serving.

Beyond the basics: *Replace the water with low-sodium vegetable broth or chicken broth for extra flavor.*

Per Serving: Calories: 260; Total fat: 8g; Carbohydrates: 39g; Fiber: 5g; Protein: 8g; Sodium: 561mg

Black Beans with Garlic and Cumin

SERVES 3 OR 4 / ACTIVE TIME: 20 MINUTES

DAIRY-FREE, GLUTEN-FREE, NUT-FREE, VEGETARIAN

For some, black beans are considered a superfood. They are filled with phytochemicals that protect your cells from damage, which, in turn, is thought to help prevent cancer. Black beans are also packed with lots of antioxidants. They are a great source of fiber and protein and when paired with Southwest-Style Quinoa (page 25) make for a complete meal.

1⅓ cups dried black beans

½ yellow onion, chopped

2 garlic cloves, minced

2 bay leaves

½ teaspoon ground cumin, plus more as needed

½ teaspoon chili powder, plus more as needed

1 teaspoon sea salt

Juice of ½ lime

1. In a colander, rinse the beans under cool running water. Discard any stones or debris.

2. Pour the beans into a medium saucepan, and cover with 2 inches of fresh water (better to add too much than not enough).

3. Add the onion, garlic, bay leaves, cumin, and chili powder. Bring to a boil over high heat. Cook for 1 minute.

4. Reduce the heat to low. Simmer for 1½ to 2 hours, or until the beans are tender. Simmer less for firmer beans and longer for creamier beans.

5. Stir in the salt and lime juice. Remove from the heat and discard the bay leaves. Taste, and add a pinch more cumin or chili powder if needed.

Make it easier: *Use 1 (15-ounce) can no-salt-added black beans, drained and rinsed, instead of dried black beans. Heat in a small pot with the onion, garlic, bay leaves, cumin, and chili powder over medium heat for 10 to 15 minutes, then follow step 5.*

Per Serving: Calories: 308; Total fat: 1g; Carbohydrates: 57g; Fiber: 14g; Protein: 19g; Sodium: 562mg

Blanch

Blanching involves placing food, usually a vegetable or fruit, into boiling water for a short amount of time—between 1 and 5 minutes—then quickly transferring it to a bowl of ice water or running it under cold water to stop the cooking process. This method is often used when preparing ingredients to be frozen, since it slows the enzymatic process that normally causes the deterioration of flavor, color, and texture. Another benefit is that it rids the food of bacteria and surface dirt, brightens the color, and slows the loss of vitamins during the cooking process.

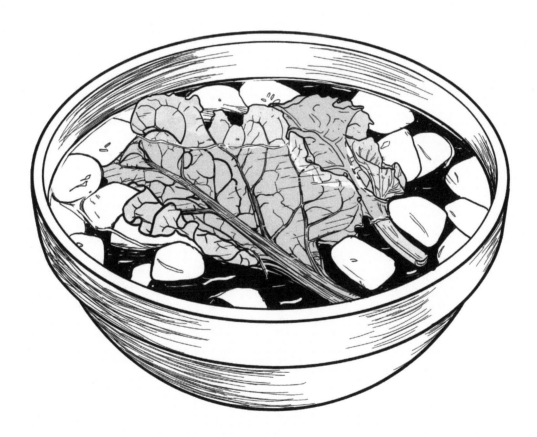

Swiss Chard Tortillas

SERVES 3 OR 4 / ACTIVE TIME: 5 MINUTES

- -

DAIRY-FREE, GLUTEN-FREE, NUT-FREE, VEGETARIAN

- -

Swiss chard is a large, colorful green leaf that can be used as a carb-free tortilla. It is rich with vitamin K, which is vital for blood regulation, bone metabolism, strength, and memory. Blanching this green also cleanses the surface of dirt and organisms and brightens the color. Wrap Southwest-Style Quinoa (page 25) and Black Beans with Garlic and Cumin (page 26) into these leaves for a tasty, ultra-healthy burrito.

4 large Swiss chard leaves   1 teaspoon sea salt

1. Rinse the chard, and cut off the thicker parts of the stems. Discard the stems, or save for another use.

2. Fill a large bowl with cold water and ice to make an ice bath.

3. Fill a large pot with water, and add the salt. Bring to a boil over high heat.

4. Put the leaves into the boiling water, and cook for 15 seconds. Remove from the heat. Drain quickly, and place the leaves into the ice bath to stop the cooking and cool. Remove the leaves, and squeeze out any excess liquid.

5. Line a baking sheet with a clean kitchen towel.

6. Arrange the leaves in a single layer on the towel, and let cool completely. Use like a tortilla, and stuff with your favorite wrap and burrito fillings.

Healthy swap: *Replace the chard with spinach and cook similarly, or use kale and collard greens, boiling them for 2 minutes instead of 15 seconds.*

Per Serving: Calories: 12; Total fat: 0g; Carbohydrates: 2g; Fiber: 1g; Protein: 1g; Sodium: 679mg

Steam

Steaming is another simple, healthy way to cook vegetables, using the heat from the boiling water without adding oil or fat (as with sautéing, roasting, or grilling). It also avoids cooking out any beneficial nutrients (as boiling directly in water can do), and it makes foods easier to digest.

To steam, fill a pot with water about one-fourth full, place a steamer basket in the pot above the water, and bring the water to a boil. Put your ingredients into the basket, cover the pot with a lid, and let them cook in the steam. If steaming in a microwave, put your ingredient into a microwave-safe bowl and add 2 to 3 tablespoons of water. Cover the bowl tightly, and microwave on high power for 3 to 4 minutes. A few types of vegetables great for steaming are artichokes, broccoli, Brussels sprouts, carrots, green beans, and turnips. Fish is also great to steam, keeping it as light and digestible as possible. No fats or oils need to be added, and the lower temperature of steaming helps preserve the beneficial omega-3 fatty acids better than other cooking methods.

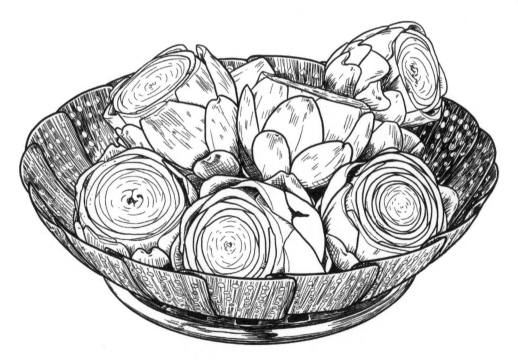

Lemon Artichokes with Dijon Yogurt Dip

SERVES 3 OR 4 / ACTIVE TIME: 10 MINUTES

- -

GLUTEN-FREE, NUT-FREE, VEGETARIAN

- -

Artichoke is a fun finger food but needs to be cooked thoroughly, or it can be tough and prickly! It is full of inulin, a unique form of fiber known to boost your immune system and help with the absorption of minerals such as calcium. Some even say it helps reduce and cure allergies! This recipe is an easy and delicious appetizer.

4 medium artichokes

1 lemon, halved

1 cup plain, full-fat Greek yogurt

1 tablespoon Dijon mustard

Coarse sea salt

1. Prepare the artichokes for steaming by snapping off the tougher outer leaves. Using a serrated knife, cut off the top third of each artichoke. Cut off the bottom stems so the artichokes stand up.

2. Use a lemon half to rub the cut surfaces of each artichoke to prevent discoloration.

3. Set a steamer basket in a large pot, and fill the pot with water, making sure the water reaches just below the basket. Bring to a boil over high heat.

4. Place the artichokes, stem-side up, in the steamer basket. Cover the pot, and steam for about 35 minutes, or until you can easily pierce the bottom of an artichoke with a knife. Remove from the heat.

5. While the artichokes steam, to make the dip, in a small bowl, stir together the yogurt and mustard.

6. Add the juice of the remaining lemon half, and stir to combine. Taste, and season with salt if needed.

7. Serve the whole artichokes with the dip on the side. To eat, remove the leaves with your fingers, and dip each leaf into the yogurt. Scrape off the meat from the leaves with your teeth.

Beyond the basics: *Add ½ teaspoon curry powder to the dip for a kick!*

Per Serving: Calories: 154; Total fat: 3g; Carbohydrates: 27g; Fiber: 12g; Protein: 10g; Sodium: 350mg

Poach

Poaching is a gentle way to cook delicate ingredients such as eggs, fish, and poultry. To poach, bring a pot of water to a boil, then reduce the heat to a simmer. Depending on the ingredients you're cooking with, you may need to turn the heat down even more. The water should be hot, but not at a rolling boil. When an egg is poached, it's gently placed into the water without the shell, so the water needs to be at a relatively low temperature so the egg is not tossed around or broken apart by powerful bubbles.

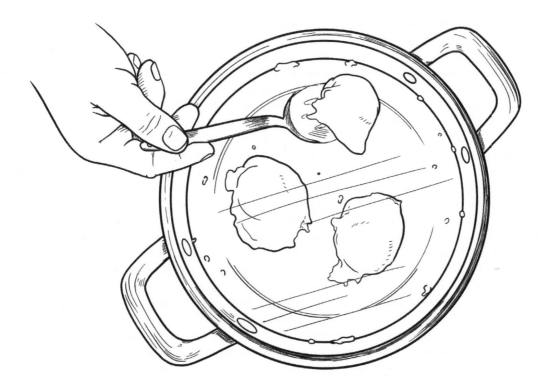

Poached Eggs with Summer Tomatoes

SERVES 4 / ACTIVE TIME: 15 MINUTES

DAIRY-FREE, NUT-FREE

Poached eggs are often enjoyed for their supple exterior and runny, sauce-like interior. This is my favorite way to eat eggs. Eggs are full of omega-3s, which contribute to brain health as well as hair and nail strength. If tomatoes are in season, the flavors of this dish work brilliantly and make for a delicious protein- and fiber-rich breakfast.

Sea salt

2 tomatoes, preferably heirloom

1 tablespoon extra-virgin olive oil

4 sourdough bread slices

4 large eggs

Pinch freshly ground black pepper

1. Fill a medium pot with about 2 inches of water, and add 1 teaspoon of salt. Bring to a boil.

2. Meanwhile, fill a medium bowl with water and ice to make an ice bath.

3. Using a serrated knife, cut the tomatoes into 8 slices, and sprinkle each with salt.

4. Drizzle the oil onto the bread, and toast in a toaster or in a preheated 425°F oven until lightly browned and crunchy.

5. Layer 2 tomato slices on each piece of toast.

6. Reduce the heat to medium. Bring the boiling water to a simmer.

7. Crack each egg into a small bowl. One at a time and working quickly, carefully submerge each bowl with an egg into the simmering water, and slide the egg into the water.

8. Turn off the heat. Immediately cover the pot. Let the eggs sit for 5 minutes to poach.

9. Using a slotted spoon, remove the eggs from the hot water, and dunk them into the ice bath.

10. Put 1 egg on top of each piece of toast. Sprinkle a little salt and pepper on each egg. Eat immediately, letting the runny yolk ooze onto the fresh tomato.

Beyond the basics: *Add avocado slices for an extra layer of creamy deliciousness.*

Per Serving: Calories: 286; Total fat: 10g; Carbohydrates: 36g; Fiber: 2g; Protein: 14g; Sodium: 498mg

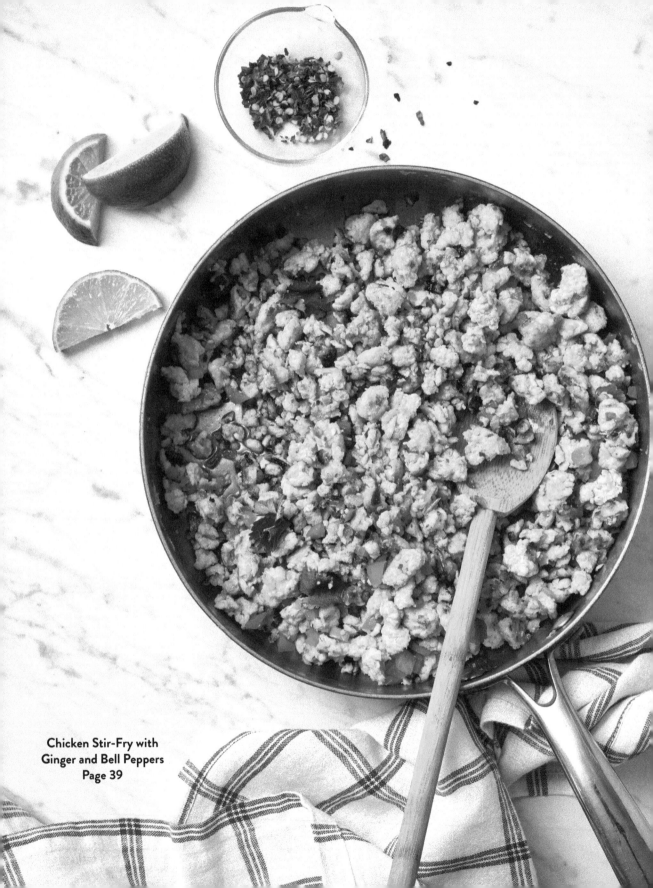

**Chicken Stir-Fry with
Ginger and Bell Peppers
Page 39**

CHAPTER FOUR

PAN COOKING

- - - - -

In this chapter, you'll learn the variations of pan cooking—how most people envision a chef whipping up dinner in the kitchen, multiple pans going, flames roaring. You'll practice with a variety of recipes that exemplify frying, sautéing, and stir-frying to make you a pro.

How to Fry Light

When using a pan to cook, it's easy to control the amount of oil or fat used. Most recipes start with a couple tablespoons of olive oil, but you can adjust the amount to your liking. Like most cooking, start with the heat high, so the pan and oil become very hot. Depending on what you're cooking, afterward you may keep the heat at medium or bring it down to low. Stir the food often if the heat is high, to keep it from burning. Give the pan a little shake, too, to spread out the contents evenly in the pan. When browning, like when caramelizing onions, bring the heat to low, and let them cook slowly and steadily, stirring every now and again to keep them from burning.

Sauté

Sautéing is a relatively quick way to cook, usually over high heat, that uses a little oil or fat in a pan. In French, *sauter* literally means "to jump." Don't be alarmed if your onions jump out of the hot pan, as if dancing. There are many ingredients that can be sautéed—vegetables, such as carrots, celery, chard, kale, onion, and spinach; meats, such as beef rib eye, pork tenderloin, and chicken breasts; fish, such as salmon and various white fishes; and shellfish, such as shrimp and scallops. When sautéing, you want the heat to be fairly high, so watch your food to make sure it doesn't burn.

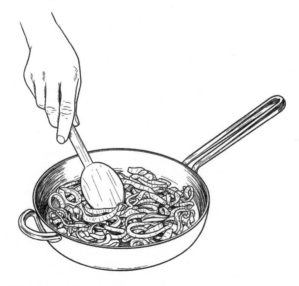

Sautéed Onions

Try It: Sauté

SERVES 4 / ACTIVE TIME: 20 MINUTES

- -

DAIRY-FREE, GLUTEN-FREE, NUT-FREE, VEGETARIAN

- -

Onions are a staple in most recipes, contributing tons of flavor and aroma. I use them in almost all dishes I cook, especially because they have antibacterial properties that help my body fight off potential illness. In this recipe, we give them a light caramelization, resulting in a sweet flavor and caramel color. They can be served alongside any type of protein, mixed into a stir-fry, used as a low-fat alternative to cheese to top a burger, or included as a flavor boost on Grilled Tri-Tip with Chimichurri (page 131).

2 large yellow or red onions

2 tablespoons extra-virgin olive oil

¼ cup balsamic vinegar, red wine, white wine, chicken stock, vegetable stock, or water

½ teaspoon sea salt, plus more as needed

1. Halve the onions from root to stem. Place the halves, cut-side down, on a cutting board, and cut them in half against the grain. Pull off the outer layer (sometimes 2 layers), and discard. Thinly slice the onions into half-moons.

2. Preheat a large pan over medium-high heat for about 30 seconds, or until hot.

3. Pour in the oil, and add the onions. Shake the pan to spread them out. Cook for 2 to 3 minutes. Stir to coat all the onions with the oil.

4. Reduce the heat to medium. Cook, stirring every 5 minutes or so with a wooden spoon and scraping up any browned bits on the bottom of the pan to avoid burning, for 10 minutes. The onions will start to soften and turn translucent. They should release liquid into the pan. Continue cooking, stirring occasionally, for 5 to 10 minutes more, or until the onions become golden brown and jammy.

5. Stir in the vinegar and salt, and deglaze the pan by scraping up any browned bits on the bottom. Let the liquid soak into the onions. Taste, and add more salt as you like. Remove from the heat. Serve hot.

Beyond the basics: *Add 2 teaspoons dried herbs or 2 tablespoons fresh herbs, minced, such as basil, oregano, rosemary, or thyme.*

Per Serving: Calories: 104; Total fat: 7g; Carbohydrates: 10g; Fiber: 1g; Protein: 1g; Sodium: 152mg

Stir-Fry

Stir-frying is a form of cooking originating in China. Similar to sautéing, stir-frying involves cooking ingredients with a bit of hot oil or fat briskly over high heat. As the name suggests, you stir the food regularly, since this is a quick and hot cooking process. Stir-fry is perfect for mixing proteins and vegetables to create a wholesome meal quickly. Mix any type of protein with vegetables such as snap peas, bell peppers, carrots, onions, ginger, and garlic.

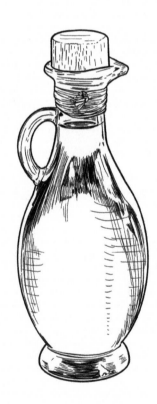

Chicken Stir-Fry with Ginger and Bell Peppers

Try It: Stir-Fry

SERVES 4 / ACTIVE TIME: 20 MINUTES

DAIRY-FREE, GLUTEN-FREE, NUT-FREE

When choosing chicken, I recommend ground chicken breast as the healthiest option. It is a very lean protein with minimal fat and great for helping your muscles recover. Even more beneficial, ginger may help with arthritis and inflammation, and the bell peppers will pump you with vitamins A and C, keeping the immune system strong. This recipe is sweet with a kick and will leave you feeling your best.

1 tablespoon extra-virgin olive oil

½ yellow onion, coarsely chopped

1 red, yellow, or green bell pepper, diced

1 teaspoon minced peeled fresh ginger

2 pounds ground chicken breast

½ cup low-sodium chicken broth

½ teaspoon sea salt, plus pinch

½ teaspoon cumin

½ teaspoon red pepper flakes

Juice of ¼ lime

½ cup cilantro leaves

1. Preheat a large pan over medium-high heat for about 30 seconds, or until hot.

2. Pour in the oil, and add the onion. Cook for about 3 minutes, or until the onion starts to caramelize and turn translucent in spots.

3. Stir in the bell pepper. Cook for 3 minutes, or until slightly soft and starting to brown.

4. Stir in the ginger and chicken. Cook for 3 to 5 minutes, or until the chicken browns.

5. Pour the chicken broth over the chicken and add the salt, cumin, and red pepper flakes. Cook, stirring, for 3 to 5 minutes, or until the chicken is thoroughly cooked and no longer pink, and the liquid has been absorbed.

6. Add the lime juice. Taste, and add a pinch more salt if needed. Remove from the heat. Serve hot, garnished with the cilantro.

Beyond the basics: *Add 2 minced garlic cloves with the ginger for a whole new level of flavor.*

Per Serving: Calories: 373; Total fat: 22g; Carbohydrates: 5g; Fiber: 1g; Protein: 40g; Sodium: 312mg

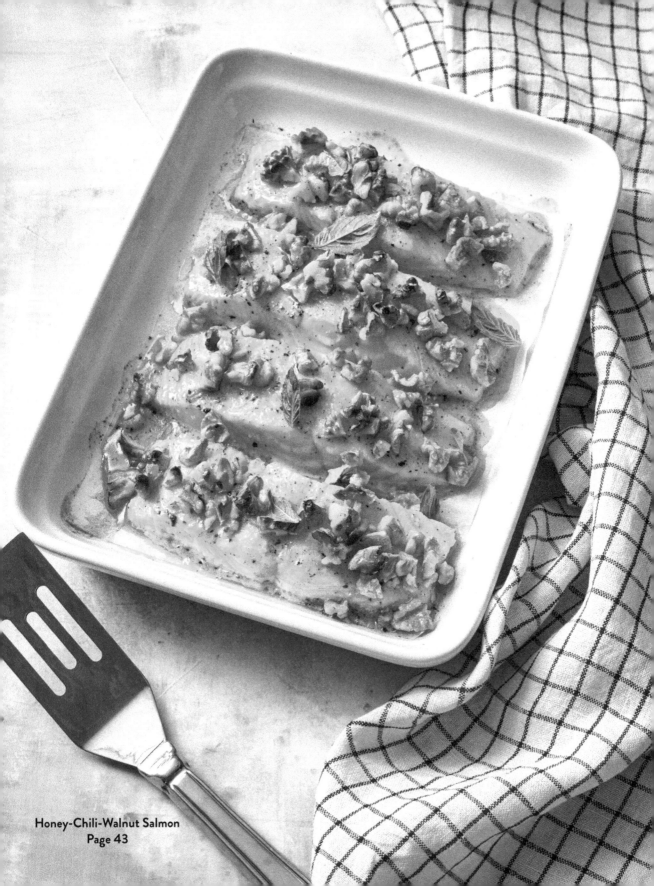

Honey-Chili-Walnut Salmon
Page 43

CHAPTER FIVE

OVEN COOKING

- - - - -

I find oven cooking to be one of the most gratifying methods of cooking. Usually, just a small amount of prep is required before you can sit back, relax, let the oven do the work, and wait for the timer to ding. In this chapter, you'll hone this skill.

How to Harness Dry Heat

Oven cooking transforms ingredients into beautifully browned, flavorful, nutrient-rich meals with minimal effort. When roasting a chicken, its exterior should become browned and crisp but it should remain tender and moist inside. Oven-cooked foods tend to be low in fat; oftentimes, just a few tablespoons of olive oil and a pinch of salt are needed to get the flavors going. Preheat the oven so the temperature is accurate before placing the ingredients inside. Also, make note of where your racks are positioned—if closer to the bottom of the oven, foods may cook faster (and slower toward the top). In some cases, this may be desirable, as when roasting potatoes to become super crispy. Place your rack in the middle position for more even cooking.

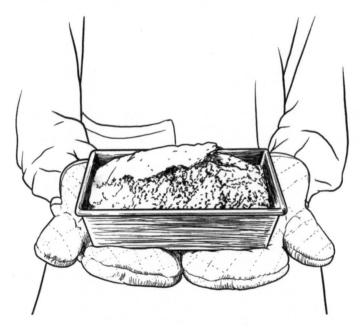

Bake

Baking is a method of cooking, usually in an oven, that uses dry heat, which slowly transfers from the outside to the inside of the food, allowing for relatively even cooking. Certain types of foods suitable for baking include fish (such as salmon), breads, tarts (both savory and sweet), quiche, cookies, cakes, pies, loaves, and many other sweet *baked* goods.

Honey-Chili-Walnut Salmon

Try It: Bake

SERVES 3 OR 4 / ACTIVE TIME: 15 MINUTES

DAIRY-FREE, GLUTEN-FREE

Passed down from my aunt, Chef Kristie, I often make this recipe when guests come for dinner. Rich in omega-3s, it is great for your hair and nails. Note: Letting the salmon rest after cooking is key to allowing the juices and flavor soak in.

2 tablespoons extra-virgin olive oil

2 tablespoons runny honey

⅛ teaspoon chili powder

1 pound skinless salmon fillets, cut into 4 even pieces

½ teaspoon fine sea salt

½ teaspoon freshly ground black pepper

2 cups chopped raw walnuts

1. Preheat the oven to 400°F. Line a 9-by-9-inch casserole dish with a 9-by-9-inch square piece of parchment paper.

2. In a small bowl, whisk together the oil, honey, and chili powder to blend.

3. Arrange the salmon pieces in the prepared dish, leaving some space between each. Sprinkle with the salt and pepper.

4. Drizzle the honey mixture all over the salmon.

5. Sprinkle the salmon with the walnuts.

6. Transfer the casserole dish to the oven, and bake, uncovered, for 9 to 12 minutes, or until the salmon has *just* cooked through (about 145°F; if you like your fish undercooked, cook until it is at least above 110°F) and the walnuts are slightly brown but not burnt. You can cut into the middle of a piece of salmon; it should no longer be dark pink and raw, but light pink. Remove from the oven. Cover with aluminum foil, and let rest for 5 minutes.

Beyond the basics: *Serving this to guests? From a bunch of fresh basil, select 5 large leaves, and stack them. Roll the leaves into a cigar-like formation. Hold the roll firmly at one end, and thinly slice across the roll, "chiffonade"-style. Sprinkle the basil leaf strands over the cooked salmon to add another layer of flavor and to beautify your creation.*

Per Serving: Calories: 847; Total fat: 69g; Carbohydrates: 22g; Fiber: 5g; Protein: 42g; Sodium: 305mg

Zucchini Loaf

SERVES 12 / ACTIVE TIME: 15 MINUTES

GLUTEN-FREE, VEGETARIAN

The ingredients in this recipe make for a hearty, healthy, tasty version of banana bread that uses zucchini instead. Zucchini adds a nice texture, and you'll hardly taste it since it is composed mostly of water.

6 tablespoons coconut oil, melted, plus more for the pan

2¼ cups gluten-free 1:1 flour, plus more for the pan

3 large eggs, at room temperature

1½ cups milk of choice

1 cup grated zucchini

¾ cup maple syrup

1 tablespoon baking powder

¼ teaspoon fine sea salt

1. Preheat the oven to 350°F. Coat the bottom and sides of a 9-by-5-inch bread loaf pan with oil. Sprinkle a bit of flour over the oil, and shake the pan to coat all sides. Knock out any excess flour.

2. In a medium bowl, using a whisk or electric mixer, beat the eggs.

3. Using a wooden spoon, stir in the milk, oil, zucchini, and maple syrup.

4. In another medium bowl, stir together the flour, baking powder, and salt.

5. To make the batter, add the dry ingredients to the zucchini mixture, and using a wooden spoon, stir until combined and smooth. Do not overmix.

6. Pour the batter into the prepared loaf pan, and using a spoon or spatula, spread it out, smoothing the top.

7. Transfer the loaf pan to the oven, and bake for 50 minutes to 1 hour, or until a toothpick or knife inserted into the center comes out clean. Be careful not to over-cook the loaf. Remove from the oven. Let sit for at least 10 minutes before slicing.

Beyond the basics: *Mix in 1 teaspoon vanilla extract and 1 teaspoon ground cinnamon for extra flavor. Other additions that taste great in this bread are 1 cup chopped nuts, such as walnuts or pecans, and 1 cup dark chocolate chunks.*

Per Serving: Calories: 235; Total fat: 9g; Carbohydrates: 34g; Fiber: 1g; Protein: 5g; Sodium: 84mg

Roast

Roasting transforms simple ingredients into something delicious, vibrant, and elegant. Very often when roasting, ingredients are mixed with a few tablespoons of olive oil and some salt, then placed into a baking dish, such as Pyrex brand, or on a stainless-steel baking sheet. Specialty roasting pans are not necessary to achieve great results. You can add whatever flair or flavor your heart desires.

When roasting meat, massage it with salt and pepper beforehand so they seep into the tissues. With chicken specifically, salt rubbed onto the skin helps transform it into a golden, crispy exterior once roasted. Many foods can be roasted: meats, such as beef, chicken, lamb, and pork; fish, like branzino, halibut, and salmon; vegetables, especially tougher root vegetables like beets, carrots, parsnips, potatoes, rutabaga, squash varieties, and sweet potatoes; some green vegetables, which cook more quickly, such as asparagus, broccoli, Brussels sprouts, and green beans; and mushrooms.

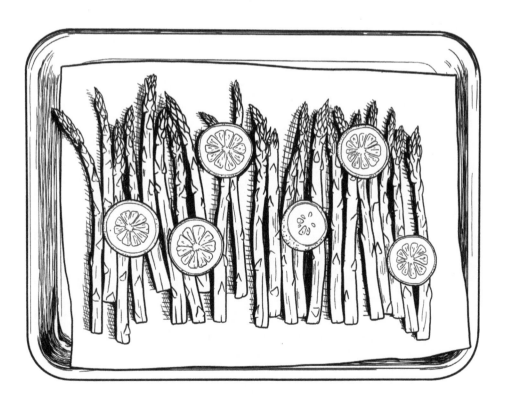

Roasted Lemon Asparagus with Crunchy Almonds

SERVES 2 / ACTIVE TIME: 15 MINUTES

DAIRY-FREE, GLUTEN-FREE, VEGETARIAN

A springtime staple, asparagus is a nutritious vegetable that only takes a little bit of work to make delicious. This simple asparagus pairs well with the Honey-Chili-Walnut Salmon recipe (page 43). Make sure to watch the asparagus while it cooks because it cooks fast!

8 ounces or 1 bunch thick asparagus, rinsed

2 large garlic cloves, peeled and minced

½ teaspoon sea salt

½ teaspoon freshly ground black pepper

2 tablespoons extra-virgin olive oil

1 tablespoon freshly squeezed lemon juice

Pinch cayenne pepper

1 cup slivered almonds

1. Preheat the oven to 425°F. Line a baking sheet with parchment paper.

2. Snap each asparagus spear at the natural breaking point, which is usually about halfway up. Discard the bottoms, which are not very edible.

3. In a large bowl, combine the asparagus, garlic, salt, pepper, oil, lemon juice, and cayenne. Toss to coat.

4. Using tongs, place the asparagus side by side on the prepared baking sheet.

5. Transfer the baking sheet to the oven, and roast for 12 to 15 minutes, or until the asparagus is tender inside and brown and crispy outside. Remove from the oven.

6. Sprinkle with the almonds. Serve immediately.

Beyond the basics: *Preheat a grill to between 450°F and 500°F. Follow steps 2 through 3. Using tongs, place the asparagus side by side on the hot grill, and close the lid. Grill for 3 to 5 minutes, or until the bottom side of the asparagus is golden brown. Using tongs, rotate the asparagus to cook the opposite side for about 3 minutes more, or until tender inside and brown and crispy outside. (Total cook time is shorter because the temperature here is higher.) Keep an eye on the asparagus, especially when thin; they cook quickly.*

Per Serving: Calories: 461; Total fat: 41g; Carbohydrates: 18g; Fiber: 9g; Protein: 14g; Sodium: 352mg

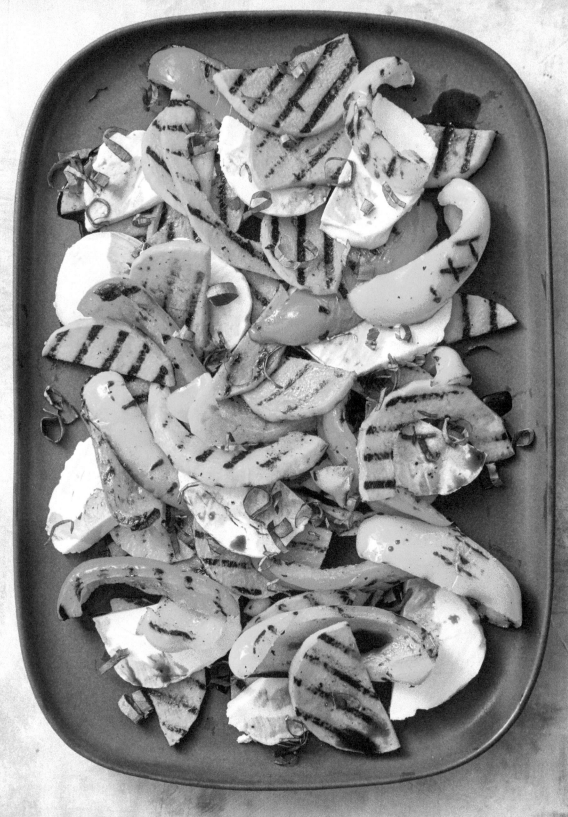

Blistered Bell Pepper and
Butternut Squash Antipasti
Page 53

CHAPTER SIX

GRILLING

- - - - -

Grilling over an open flame—watching ingredients transform from raw to tender in front of your eyes—brings ultimate satisfaction at an almost primal level. Grilling involves cooking food quickly with direct or indirect dry heat, so it requires extra attention. It is most often used for cooking meats, fish, and vegetables.

How to Harness Direct Heat

Even if you've never attempted grilling, it's not as tricky as you might think. Grilled meats are often lower in fat, since excess fat drips off while cooking. Vegetables can be placed straight on the grill, just as they are, to let the open flame do the work of creating a delicious char on the skin.

Stovetop Grill Pans

Stovetop grill pans are convenient and easy to use. Simply place the pan over your gas or electric burner, and bring the heat to high. Once the pan is hot, lower the heat slightly, and place your ingredients on the pan so the food gets a nice sear. Be sure to keep watch to prevent burning, and turn the ingredients once they are a dark brown color on the cooked side.

Gas + Charcoal Grills

Gas and charcoal grills require cooking outside on a deck, in the backyard, or in a public park with such facilities. When cooking with direct heat, you put the food right over the fire. This method is great for fast-cooking vegetables and thin cuts of meats. Using indirect heat means placing food farther away from the fire and is more suitable for a slower cooking process.

When using a charcoal grill, set up the coals to your liking, so there is either direct or indirect heat (or both). Light the coals at least 20 minutes before cooking. Pour enough charcoal into the grill to make the layers needed. Stack the charcoal into an upside-down cone shape. Pour lighter fluid on the charcoal cone, primarily in the center, and let it soak in for at least 30 seconds. Use about ¼ cup of fluid for each pound of charcoal. Starting on the bottom of at least two sides, light the charcoal. Let the coals burn until all of them appear white on the surface. Using a long pair of tongs, spread the coals across the bottom of the grill. Close the lid, and wait at least 5 minutes for the heat to build. Open the lid, add the food, and start cooking!

Gas grills are straightforward: turn on the gas, and press the ignitor button to light the grill. With strong, direct heat, ingredients cook quickly on the outside, but the heat may not transfer to the inside before the outside becomes burnt. Lessen the strength of the heat, or move the food farther away from the heat if it requires a slightly slower, more even cooking process.

Proteins

When grilling meats and plant-based proteins, you'll want a fairly strong heat. Once the food is cooked on one side, reduce the heat slightly and flip to cook the other side. A few foods perfect for grilling include beef steaks, burgers (animal- or plant-based), chicken legs, lamb chops, pork ribs, salmon, sausage, and shrimp.

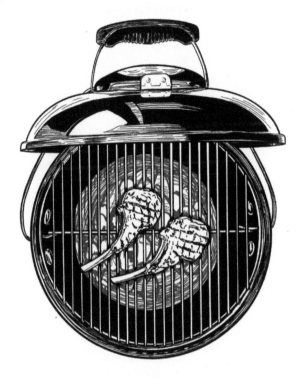

Vegetables

Depending on the vegetables you're grilling, you may want to grill them whole, halved, or in long strips. Some favorites to grill include larger vegetables such as zucchini, bell peppers, and eggplant. Brush them with a bit of olive oil and sprinkle with salt before placing them on the grill. Let them char slightly all around the outer skin. Other vegetables perfect for grilling include asparagus, corn, mushrooms, onions, shishito peppers, squash, and tomatoes.

Rosemary Lamb Chops

SERVES 4 / ACTIVE TIME: 20 MINUTES

DAIRY-FREE, GLUTEN-FREE, NUT-FREE

Lamb is incredibly rich in protein, vitamins, and minerals. It also tends to be leaner and more tender than beef or pork. If it is fresh, it shouldn't taste too "lamb-y." That flavor develops as the meat sits. Rosemary and lamb are a classic combination, creating a delicious flavor and aroma reminiscent of Mediterranean cuisine.

2 tablespoons olive oil

2 tablespoons fresh rosemary leaves, chopped, or 2 teaspoons dried (fresh is recommended)

3 or 4 garlic cloves, minced

½ teaspoon sea salt

½ teaspoon freshly ground black pepper

2 pounds lamb chops

1. In a medium casserole dish, stir together the oil, rosemary, garlic, salt, and pepper.

2. Add the lamb chops, and using your hands, rub the seasoning over the chops. Cover the dish, and refrigerate to marinate for at least 2 hours, flipping the chops and rubbing the seasoning over them every 30 minutes, or overnight, if possible. Remove from the refrigerator 1 hour before cooking.

3. Preheat a grill on high heat until it reaches at least 500°F.

4. Reduce the heat to medium. Put the lamb chops on the grill directly over the heat. Cook for 4 minutes, or until dark grill marks appear.

5. Flip the chops, and cook for 3 minutes, or until dark grill marks appear on the other side.

6. Turn off one of the burners, and move the chops to that (cooler) side, so they are now over indirect heat. Cook for 2 to 3 minutes more, or until just cooked through (about 145°F, or leave rare, if that is your preference). Using a knife, cut into the middle of a chop to see how much has cooked through.

7. Turn off the heat. Remove the chops from the grill, cover, and let rest for 5 to 10 minutes so the meat has time to reabsorb all the juices. Remember, the meat continues to cook after removing it from the heat, so be careful not to overcook it.

Per Serving: Calories: 766; Total fat: 67g; Carbohydrates: 1g; Fiber: 0g; Protein: 37g; Sodium: 360mg

Blistered Bell Pepper and Butternut Squash Antipasti

SERVES 4 / ACTIVE TIME: 20 MINUTES

- -

GLUTEN-FREE, NUT-FREE, VEGETARIAN

- -

Grilled bell peppers are one of the easiest, most delicious sweet snacks to make. They also happen to be an excellent source of vitamins A and C, potassium, and fiber. But beware—bell peppers are part of a plant group known as nightshades, which can trigger inflammatory reactions in some people. Other types of night-shades include cayenne pepper, eggplant, potatoes, and tomatoes. Paprika, which comes from peppers, can also cause problems. If you have sensitivities to nightshades, certainly avoid them. Otherwise, they are a nutritious category of vegetables and fruits to include in your healthy diet.

Leaves from 1 bunch fresh basil

1 red bell pepper

1 yellow bell pepper

1 butternut squash

1 recipe SPOOG (page 18)

1 (8-ounce) ball fresh mozzarella cheese, cut into rounds

2 tablespoons balsamic vinegar

1. Rinse and dry the basil leaves. Stack the leaves, and roll them like a cigar. Thinly slice across the roll, cutting the basil into long thin strands.

2. Remove the stem and seeds from the red and yellow bell peppers, then cut each into 8 long, thick slices. Transfer to a large bowl.

3. Using a knife or vegetable peeler, peel the butternut squash. Halve it length-wise. Using a spoon, scoop out the seeds and membranes, and discard. Place the squash halves, cut-side down, on a work surface, and cut them into ¼-inch half-moons. Add to the bowl with the peppers.

4. Add the SPOOG, and toss to coat.

5. Preheat a grill on medium-high heat.

>>

6. When the grill is hot, reduce the heat to medium. Arrange the vegetables next to each other on the grill. Keep an eye on them so they do not burn. Cook the bell peppers for about 8 minutes, or until dark grill marks are clear. Flip, and cook for 5 minutes, or until the other side has grill marks. Cook the butternut squash for about 10 minutes, or until tender. Flip, and cook for 8 minutes on the second side. Remove from the heat.

7. Arrange the cooked vegetables on a serving platter in a pleasing design.

8. Randomly place the cheese slices on top.

9. Drizzle with the vinegar, and sprinkle with the basil. Serve hot or at room temperature.

Healthy swap: *Skip the mozzarella if you want to make this dairy-free.*

Per Serving: Calories: 304; Total fat: 16g; Carbohydrates: 27g; Fiber: 5g; Protein: 15g; Sodium: 541mg

3

HEALTHY RECIPES TO
BRING IT ALL TOGETHER

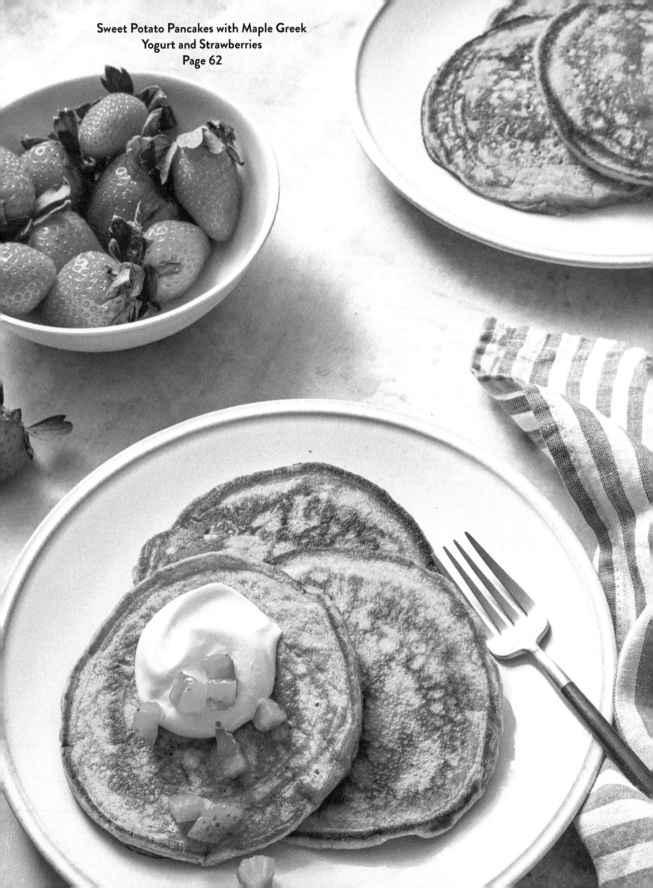

Sweet Potato Pancakes with Maple Greek
Yogurt and Strawberries
Page 62

CHAPTER SEVEN

BREAKFAST

- - - - -

Mom's Cinnamon-Walnut Granola

SERVES 4 / ACTIVE TIME: 20 MINUTES

GLUTEN-FREE, VEGETARIAN

My mom ate cereal or granola for breakfast every day. When I was old enough to cook, I made homemade granola and added tons of cinnamon. She loved it! I always add cinnamon now and think of her. Cinnamon is full of antioxidants and is also anti-inflammatory. Walnuts add protein as well as crunch.

1½ cups rolled oats

1 cup unsweetened coconut flakes

½ cup walnuts, coarsely chopped

½ cup chia seeds, flaxseed, sesame seeds, or poppy seeds

¼ cup coconut oil

¼ cup maple syrup

¼ cup cocoa powder

2 teaspoons ground cinnamon

1 teaspoon vanilla extract

½ teaspoon fine sea salt

Milk or plain Greek yogurt, for serving

1. Preheat the oven to 350°F. Line a baking sheet with parchment paper.

2. In a large bowl, stir together the oats, coconut flakes, walnuts, and seeds.

3. In a small saucepan, melt the oil over medium-low heat.

4. Whisk the maple syrup, cocoa powder, cinnamon, vanilla, and salt into the saucepan. Remove from the heat.

5. Pour the liquid ingredients over the dry ingredients, and fold to coat.

6. Spread the mixture onto the prepared baking sheet, and using the back of a spatula, press firmly into an even layer to ensure that the mixture is compact.

7. Transfer the baking sheet to the oven, and bake for 15 to 20 minutes. Remove from the oven. Flip the granola in large chunks, and bake for 10 minutes more, stirring every 3 to 4 minutes, or until toasted and fragrant. The darker color makes it hard to tell if it is cooked, so go by smell, or taste a walnut to see if it is cooked. It should be nutty and pleasantly roasted. Remove from the oven. Let cool completely.

8. Serve the granola at room temperature in milk or on top of plain Greek yogurt.

Healthy swap: *If you want less sugar, reduce the amount of maple syrup by half.*

Per Serving: Calories: 643; Total fat: 42g; Carbohydrates: 60g; Fiber: 19g; Protein: 15g; Sodium: 188mg

Tricked Out Overnight Oats

SERVES 12 / ACTIVE TIME: 5 MINUTES

GLUTEN-FREE, VEGETARIAN

This is a fun and super easy grab-and-go breakfast—it just needs to be prepared the night before. The seeds and nuts make it rich with protein, which stimulates the brain and the muscles. My great friend Liz, who grew up in Switzerland, taught me this classic Swiss recipe that we now love and eat often.

3 cups rolled oats

1 cup toasted almonds

1 cup unsweetened raisins or chopped dried apricots

½ cup golden flaxseed

1 cup pumpkin seeds or any seed you prefer

1 teaspoon ground cinnamon

1 teaspoon vanilla extract

2 cups plain Greek yogurt or almond milk yogurt

1 cup almond milk, plus more as needed

Fresh fruit, for serving

½ cup coconut flakes (optional)

1. In a large bowl, mix together the oats, almonds, raisins, flaxseed, pumpkin seeds, and cinnamon.

2. Add the vanilla and yogurt. Mix until it makes a pretty dense mixture.

3. Pour in the almond milk, mix, and let sit overnight, covered, in the refrigerator. If dry the next day, add another ½ cup of almond milk until it has a slightly wet consistency.

4. Serve the oats cold with fresh fruit and the coconut flakes (if using) on top.

Make it healthier: *Add an extra layer of protein by mixing in ½ cup creamy almond butter.*

Per Serving: Calories: 347; Total fat: 17g; Carbohydrates: 38g; Fiber: 8g; Protein: 14g; Sodium: 37mg

Sweet Potato Pancakes with Maple Greek Yogurt and Strawberries

SERVES 4 / ACTIVE TIME: 35 MINUTES

VEGETARIAN

Sweet potato naturally adds a creamy, rich texture to baked goods. It is also rich with nutrients, including antioxidants, which protect your body from DNA-damaging free radicals that can cause major inflammation. You can make the pancake batter a day ahead; just preheat the pan and pour the batter in when you're ready to eat!

1 cup plain, low-fat Greek yogurt, plus more for serving

4 tablespoons maple syrup, divided

2 teaspoons vanilla extract, divided

Pinch fine sea salt, plus 1½ teaspoons

1½ cups all-purpose flour or gluten-free 1:1 flour, sifted

2 teaspoons baking powder

2 teaspoons pumpkin pie spice

3 large eggs

1 cup milk of choice

3 tablespoons coconut oil, melted, plus more for cooking

1 (14-ounce) can unsweetened sweet potato puree (or pumpkin, if available)

1 cup fresh strawberries, coarsely chopped

1. In a small bowl, whisk together the yogurt, 3 tablespoons of maple syrup, 1 teaspoon of vanilla, and a pinch of salt to combine.

2. To make the batter, in a large bowl, stir together the flour, baking powder, pumpkin pie spice, and the salt.

3. In a medium bowl, whisk together the eggs, milk, oil, remaining 1 teaspoon of vanilla, and remaining 1 tablespoon of maple syrup to blend.

4. Using a wooden spoon, fold the wet ingredients into the dry ingredients, and stir to combine.

5. Add the sweet potato puree, and whisk well until smooth.

6. Preheat a large skillet over medium-high heat.

7. When the skillet is hot, pour in 1 tablespoon of oil.

8. Scoop or pour ½-cup portions of the batter into the skillet (as many as will fit with room to flip). Cook for 3 to 4 minutes, or until you see bubbles in the top and the edges of the pancakes are turning brown.

9. Using a spatula, flip the pancakes. Cook for 1 to 2 more minutes, or until the bottoms are brown. Remove from the skillet, and set aside on a plate. Cover with aluminum foil to keep warm. Repeat with the remaining batter. Turn off the heat.

10. To serve, place 3 pancakes on each plate, and top with a scoop of the yogurt mixture and the strawberries.

Make it healthier: *Try using nutrient-dense flours—such as ¾ cup buckwheat flour plus ½ cup oat flour, or 1½ cups gluten-free flour—instead of all-purpose flour.*

Per Serving: Calories: 565; Total fat: 18g; Carbohydrates: 85g; Fiber: 4g; Protein: 17g; Sodium: 785mg

Poached Eggs with Avocado and Blanched Spinach

SERVES 4 / ACTIVE TIME: 20 MINUTES

DAIRY-FREE, GLUTEN-FREE, NUT-FREE, VEGETARIAN

Not only are avocados creamy and delicious, but they are also filled with beneficial nutrients, such as potassium (more than bananas), fiber, folate, and unsaturated fats. The fats in avocados are highly beneficial for hair, skin, nails, and more. Just add an egg and spinach, and you've got a full meal!

1 teaspoon sea salt, plus more as needed

1½ pounds fresh spinach or baby spinach

Freshly ground black pepper

¼ teaspoon garlic powder

1 ripe avocado

4 large eggs

4 ounces prosciutto, chopped (optional)

1. Fill a medium pot with water, and add the salt. Bring to a boil.

2. Meanwhile, rinse the spinach. Fill a large bowl with cold water.

3. When the water boils, add the spinach, stems first, and push it down to submerge it quickly. Blanch for about 40 seconds, or until the stems are flexible. Using a large slotted spoon, immediately transfer the spinach into the cold water to stop the cooking. Reserve the cooking water. Turn off the heat.

4. Using the slotted spoon, transfer the spinach to a colander to drain excess water. Reserve the ice water.

5. Toss the spinach with a pinch of salt and pepper and the garlic powder.

6. Halve the avocado, and remove the pit (see page 151). Using your knife, cut long thin slices into the avocado flesh while it is still in its skin.

7. Return the spinach cooking water to a boil.

8. When the water boils, reduce the heat to medium. Crack each egg into its own small bowl or mug, and gently slip each egg into the water. Poach for 4 minutes.

9. Using a slotted spoon, carefully remove each egg, and place in the ice water to stop the cooking.

10. Place a scoop of spinach in the middle of each of 4 plates or wide bowls.

11. Put 1 egg on top of each pile of spinach.

12. Scoop one-fourth of the avocado onto each egg. Season with salt and pepper.

13. Sprinkle each dish with the prosciutto (if using), and serve immediately.

Beyond the basics: *Begin the base layer with cooked quinoa (see page 25) under the spinach to make it a heartier meal.*

Per Serving: Calories: 202; Total fat: 13g; Carbohydrates: 13g; Fiber: 8g; Protein: 13g; Sodium: 614mg

Apple-Buckwheat Pancakes

SERVES 2 / ACTIVE TIME: 20 MINUTES

DAIRY-FREE, GLUTEN-FREE, VEGETARIAN

Buckwheat is a seed, not a wheat, and is, therefore, gluten-free. It was a staple in traditional French kitchens and has a very soft, sweet flavor, making it perfect for pancakes or crêpes. Consider topping these pancakes with fresh berries, Greek yogurt, honey, or maple syrup. Add the zest of a lemon to the batter for a refreshing flavor element that also delivers a healthy dose of calcium, magnesium, and vitamins.

¾ cup buckwheat flour

¾ cup oat flour

1 teaspoon baking powder

½ teaspoon baking soda

½ teaspoon sea salt

1 teaspoon ground cinnamon

1 cup milk of choice

2 tablespoons pure maple syrup or honey

2 large eggs

1½ tablespoons coconut oil, melted, plus 1 tablespoon

1 apple, grated

1 teaspoon vanilla extract

1. In a medium bowl, using a wooden spoon, stir together the buckwheat flour, oat flour, baking powder, baking soda, salt, and cinnamon.

2. In another medium bowl, whisk together the milk, maple syrup, eggs, oil, apple, and vanilla to combine.

3. To make the batter, combine the dry ingredients with the wet ingredients, and using a wooden spoon, gently stir until just mixed.

4. Preheat a large sauté pan or skillet over medium-high heat.

5. When the pan is hot, pour in the remaining 1 tablespoon of oil to melt.

6. Pour ½ cup of batter into the pan (it should sizzle!). Add more ½-cup portions to fit, leaving room to flip. Cook for 5 minutes, or until the edges start to brown and bubbles form on top.

7. Flip the pancakes, and cook for 2 to 3 minutes more, or until browned. Transfer to a plate. Repeat as needed for more servings. Turn off the heat.

Make it easier: *In a blender, combine all the ingredients. Blend for 10 to 15 seconds, or until smooth; do not overblend or the pancakes will be flat.*

Per Serving: Calories: 653; Total fat: 24g; Carbohydrates: 92g; Fiber: 10g; Protein: 22g; Sodium: 921mg

Lemon-Poppy Seed Muffins

SERVES 8 / ACTIVE TIME: 20 MINUTES

DAIRY-FREE, GLUTEN-FREE, VEGETARIAN

My version of the classic, these muffins are perfect as a companion to your morning coffee or tea, as an afternoon snack, or as an evening dessert. Lemon gives these muffins a refreshing citrus flavor, and the poppy seeds add texture and color. Poppy seeds also happen to be a great source of manganese, which is important in maintaining bone health and to aid blood clotting. They're rich in fiber and healthy fats, too!

4 large eggs

⅓ cup pure maple syrup

⅓ cup freshly squeezed lemon juice (1 or 2 lemons)

¼ cup melted coconut oil or avocado oil

2 teaspoons grated lemon zest

1½ teaspoons vanilla extract

2 cups almond flour

⅓ cup tapioca flour or arrowroot flour

¼ cup poppy seeds

1 teaspoon baking soda

¼ teaspoon sea salt

1. Preheat the oven to 350°F. Line 8 wells of a standard muffin tin with paper liners.

2. In a large bowl, using a wooden spoon, stir together the eggs, maple syrup, lemon juice, oil, lemon zest, and vanilla to combine.

3. In another large bowl, stir together the almond flour, tapioca flour, poppy seeds, baking soda, and salt.

4. To make the batter, slowly pour the wet ingredients into the dry ingredients, and stir together until combined. Do not overmix.

5. Evenly fill each prepared muffin well with the batter.

6. Transfer the muffin tin to the oven, and bake for 15 minutes, or until a toothpick inserted into the center of a muffin comes out clean. Remove from the oven. Serve hot or at room temperature.

Beyond the basics: *Top these muffins with a special maple-orange glaze: In a small bowl, whisk together ½ cup maple syrup, 2 tablespoons freshly squeezed orange juice, 1 teaspoon grated orange zest, and ¼ teaspoon sea salt until smooth. Pour over the muffins as soon as you pull them from the oven.*

Per Serving: Calories: 278; Total fat: 20g; Carbohydrates: 19g; Fiber: 3g; Protein: 8g; Sodium: 254mg

Pesto Scramble

SERVES 2 / ACTIVE TIME: 10 MINUTES

GLUTEN-FREE, VEGETARIAN

Pesto is a beautiful sauce that I use on everything. Fresh basil is known to be anti-inflammatory and to fight off viruses in your body. The pine nuts are super creamy when blended and are full of protein. This scramble is what I often whip up for breakfast, or even better, when I want breakfast for dinner, paired with a fresh salad, such as Sweet Pea, Goat Cheese, and Avocado Salad with Lemon Vinaigrette (page 98).

FOR THE PESTO

1 cup tightly packed fresh basil leaves

¼ cup pine nuts

2 large garlic cloves

2 tablespoons extra-virgin olive oil

½ teaspoon sea salt, plus more as needed

¼ teaspoon freshly ground black pepper, plus more as needed

Juice of ½ lemon, plus more as needed

3 tablespoons nutritional yeast (optional)

1 ounce or 3 tablespoons freshly grated parmesan cheese (optional)

FOR THE SCRAMBLED EGGS

6 large eggs

1 tablespoon milk or water

1 tablespoon extra-virgin olive oil

1 roma tomato, diced

1. **To make the pesto:** Put the basil, pine nuts, garlic, oil, salt, pepper, lemon juice, nutritional yeast (if using), and cheese (if using) in a food processor or blender. Blend until smooth. Adjust the seasoning to taste as necessary by adding salt, pepper, and lemon juice. (The pesto can be made ahead of time and refrigerated until using. Make sure to bring to room temperature before cooking.)

2. **To make the scrambled eggs:** In a medium bowl, whisk together the eggs and milk.

3. Preheat a small saucepan over medium heat.

4. When the saucepan is warm, reduce the heat to low. Drizzle in the oil.

5. Add the eggs, and wait for the edges to just barely start to set. Then, using a rubber spatula, gently push the eggs from one edge of the pan to the other. Repeat in a different direction. Continue doing this, pausing between swipes, to allow the egg to settle on the warm pan and cook, forming curds.

6. When the eggs are mostly cooked, with big fluffy folds but still slightly wet looking, add the tomato and half of the pesto. Fold the eggs and vegetables together a couple of times. Remove from the heat. Transfer to plates. Drizzle more pesto on top, and serve hot.

Beyond the basics: *Try adding other healthy vegetables, such as ½ cup chopped canned artichoke hearts or sliced mushrooms. If using sliced mushrooms, start by sautéing the mushrooms in the skillet with 1 tablespoon olive oil before lowering the heat and adding the eggs.*

Per Serving: Calories: 447; Total fat: 38g; Carbohydrates: 8g; Fiber: 2g; Protein: 20g; Sodium: 580mg

Smoked Salmon and Goat Cheese Flatbread

SERVES 3 OR 4 / ACTIVE TIME: 20 MINUTES

NUT-FREE

Salmon is rich in omega-3 fatty acids, which are essential to our health and necessary to obtain from external sources, since our body cannot create them. Goat cheese contains less lactose than cow's milk and so is easier to digest; it has fewer calories and more vitamins and minerals compared to cow's cheese and is a healthy source of probiotics.

¾ to 1 cup whole-wheat flour or gluten-free 1:1 flour

2 teaspoons baking powder

1 teaspoon sea salt, divided

1 cup plain, full-fat Greek yogurt

2 tablespoons extra-virgin olive oil

2 garlic cloves, minced

8 ounces soft goat cheese

1 teaspoon chopped fresh herbs, such as thyme, rosemary, or basil

¼ teaspoon sea salt

8 ounces smoked salmon

¼ cup fresh dill, chopped

1. In a large bowl, combine the flour, baking powder, and salt.

2. Using your hands, slowly mix in the yogurt until the flour has absorbed the yogurt and just enough yogurt is added to form a smooth ball of dough. The dough should stay together naturally, and there should not be any flour remaining.

3. Cut the dough into 4 pieces. Roll each piece into a thin, flat circle 4 to 5 inches in diameter.

4. Preheat a large skillet over medium heat.

5. When the skillet is hot, drizzle in the oil, and add the garlic. Cook for 1 minute, or until the garlic starts releasing its aroma.

6. As soon as this occurs, add 1 flatbread, and toast for 2 to 3 minutes, or until it bubbles up on one side.

7. Flip the flatbread, and cook for 2 to 3 minutes more. Transfer to a plate, and cover with a paper towel to keep it warm. Repeat with the remaining flatbreads. Turn off the heat.

8. In a small bowl, stir together the cheese, herbs, and salt.

9. Spread the goat cheese mixture onto each flatbread.

10. Arrange the smoked salmon on top, and add a sprinkle of fresh dill. Fold the flatbread in half like a sandwich, or serve open face.

Beyond the basics: *This flatbread is very versatile and can be stored at room temperature for 2 to 3 days to be used as a crust for easy pizza, sandwich wraps, or toast for breakfast.*

Per Serving: Calories: 538; Total fat: 31g; Carbohydrates: 30g; Fiber: 1g; Protein: 34g; Sodium: 1,440mg

Fresh Fig Crumble with Thyme-Honey Coconut Cream

SERVES 4 / ACTIVE TIME: 20 MINUTES

DAIRY-FREE, GLUTEN-FREE, VEGETARIAN

This beautiful crumble is laden with color, texture, and nutrients. Figs are not only beautiful fruits but are rich in minerals such as calcium, iron, magnesium, and potassium and full of antioxidants as well. Coconut is both delicious and a wonderful source of manganese, essential for bone health.

2 (13.4-ounce) cans full-fat coconut milk or coconut cream

2 cups fresh figs, halved (or plums, pears, or apples, cut into similar size)

¼ teaspoon sea salt

1 cup almond flour, plus more as needed

¼ cup coconut oil

4 tablespoons honey, divided

½ teaspoon vanilla extract

1 teaspoon fresh thyme leaves, minced

1. Refrigerate the cans of coconut milk overnight. This helps separate the coconut cream from the coconut water.

2. Preheat the oven to 375°F.

3. In a medium serving dish, toss the figs with the salt.

4. In a medium bowl, using your hands, mix together the flour, oil, 3 tablespoons of honey, and the vanilla. If the mixture is super gooey and wet, add a little more flour until it forms a firmer dough. Transfer to an 8-by-8-inch baking dish.

5. Transfer the baking dish to the oven, and bake for 15 to 20 minutes, or until the crumble starts to brown. Remove from the oven. Let cool for 5 to 10 minutes.

6. Sprinkle the crumble over the figs.

7. Remove the coconut milk from the refrigerator, and try not to shake the cans. Open the cans, and scoop the top layer of coconut cream, just until you get to the clear water, into a small bowl. Discard or consume the coconut water.

8. Carefully fold in the thyme and remaining 1 tablespoon of honey.

9. Serve the cream on the side or over the crumble.

Make it easier: *Skip the coconut cream, and substitute plain Greek yogurt.*

Per Serving: Calories: 699; Total fat: 62g; Carbohydrates: 39g; Fiber: 4g; Protein: 8g; Sodium: 172mg

Liz's Nutty Green Bowl

SERVES 2 / ACTIVE TIME: 10 MINUTES

DAIRY-FREE, GLUTEN-FREE, VEGETARIAN

Liz is a great friend of mine and the only person I have ever let make my break-fast. Breakfast is the first meal of the day, and therefore I always want it to make me feel amazing and be exactly what I want for the start of the day. And Liz is the best at it. Here is a recipe that is not only super healthy, full of greens, nuts, and healing spices, but also absolutely delicious and hearty. It is derived from one of Liz's favorite smoothies!

2 frozen bananas, peeled, plus more as needed

2 pitted dates, plus more as needed

1 tablespoon smooth unsalted almond butter

1½ cups frozen spinach

½ teaspoon ground cinnamon

1½ cups unsweetened almond milk

1 teaspoon vanilla extract

1 tablespoon brown flaxseed (optional)

½ cup raw cashews (optional)

1 handful ice (optional)

1. In a blender, combine the bananas, dates, almond butter, spinach, cinnamon, almond milk, and vanilla. If using, add the flaxseed, cashews, and ice. Blend until smooth.

2. Taste, and adjust with extra fruit if needed. Serve immediately in a bowl or a cup with a straw, spoon, or both.

Make it easier: *Soak the dates in ½ cup water overnight, strain the water, then use the soaked dates for a creamier texture. Soaked dates can also be blended into a syrup that is tasty as a sugar replacement in many dishes.*

Per Serving: Calories: 347; Total fat: 11g; Carbohydrates: 48g; Fiber: 8g; Protein: 13g; Sodium: 167mg

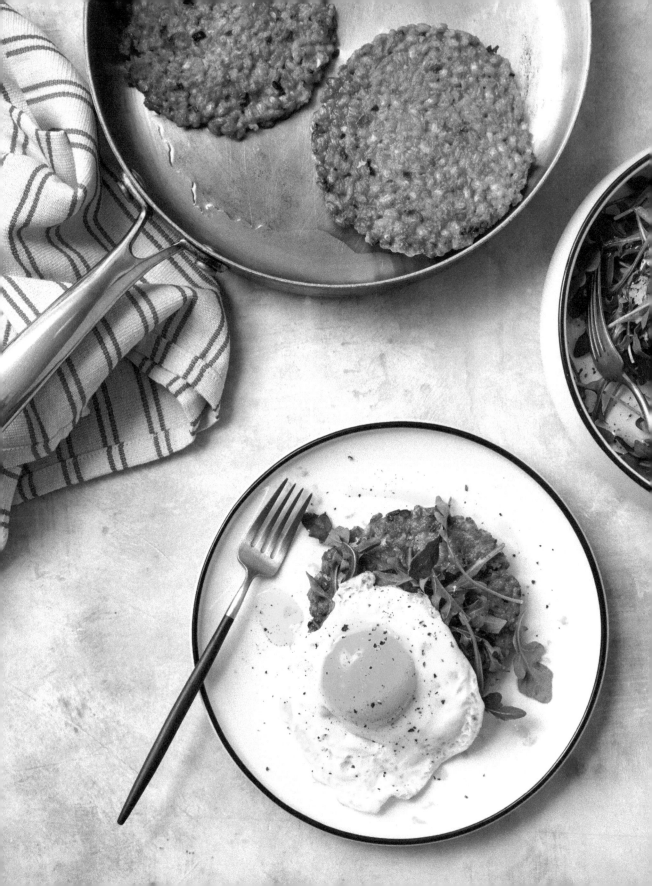

Barley Pancakes with Arugula and Sunny-Side Eggs

SERVES 4 / ACTIVE TIME: 20 MINUTES

DAIRY-FREE, NUT-FREE, VEGETARIAN

Barley was one of the earliest cultivated grains and has fed humans for centuries. It is considered healthier than rice because it is rich with fiber and calcium. However, barley is not gluten-free, unlike rice and many other grains. As the staple ingredient in this recipe, prepare for a very hearty protein- and fiber-packed healthy meal.

½ cup pearled barley

1 cup water, plus more as needed

½ teaspoon fine sea salt, plus more for the cooking water and for seasoning

¼ cup whole spelt flour or whole-wheat flour, plus more as needed

5 large eggs, 1 beaten and 4 for cooking

2 scallions, white and light green parts, thinly sliced

3 garlic cloves, minced, divided

½ serrano chile, seeded and minced

2 tablespoons olive oil, plus more for cooking the eggs and for garnish

2 cups loosely packed arugula

Juice of ½ lemon

Grated zest of ½ lemon

Freshly ground black pepper

1. In a small pot, combine the barley, water, and a few pinches of salt. Bring to a boil over high heat.

2. Once the water is boiling, reduce the heat to a simmer. Cover the pot, and cook for about 25 minutes, or until all the water has been absorbed and the barley has tripled in volume and is soft yet chewy. Remove from the heat.

3. In a large bowl, combine the cooked barley, flour, 1 beaten egg, scallions, two of the garlic cloves, the serrano chile, and ½ teaspoon of salt. Stir to combine until you have a thick, wet batter that holds together easily. If it is too wet, add a little more flour. If it is very dry, add a bit of water.

4. Divide the dough into 4 balls (about ⅓ cup each). Using wet hands, press them into wide, thin patties the size of a pancake. The patties cook better if they have had time to chill, so let them sit at least 10 minutes in the freezer or 30 minutes in the refrigerator before cooking.

5. Preheat a large skillet over medium-high heat.

>>

6. When the skillet is hot, reduce the heat to medium. Drizzle the oil into the skillet.

7. Put the pancakes into the skillet, and cook for about 5 minutes, or until they bounce back when lightly pressed and hold together when flipped.

8. Flip the pancakes, and cook the other side for 3 to 4 minutes. Transfer the pancakes to a plate, and cover with a towel to keep warm.

9. Reduce the heat to medium. Drizzle in 1 teaspoon of oil.

10. Crack the remaining 4 eggs into the skillet, spacing them evenly.

11. Reduce the heat to low. Let the eggs cook slowly for about 5 minutes, or until the whites appear completely white and no translucent parts remain. The yolks should still be runny. Remove from the heat.

12. In a medium bowl, toss the arugula with the lemon juice, lemon zest, and remaining clove of fresh minced garlic. Season with salt and pepper.

13. Place a pancake on each plate. Top each with arugula and 1 egg. Generously season with salt, pepper, and a light drizzle of oil.

Healthy swap: *Use any green, such as Swiss chard, kale, or spinach, instead of arugula, or combine a couple of options.*

Per Serving: Calories: 273; Total fat: 13g; Carbohydrates: 28g; Fiber: 5g; Protein: 12g; Sodium: 328mg

Savory Mushroom and Quinoa Porridge

SERVES 4 / ACTIVE TIME: 20 MINUTES

GLUTEN-FREE, VEGETARIAN

In this nourishing porridge that you'll want to sip on a chilly fall day, mushrooms take center stage. Mushrooms are packed with nutrients that boost the immune system, promote bone health, and help lower cholesterol, plus they're even thought to exhibit cancer-fighting properties. This porridge is a delicious, wholesome meal—quinoa being a great source of protein and fiber as well.

2 tablespoons olive oil, divided

2 medium shallots, minced

6 ounces cremini mushrooms

1 teaspoon fresh rosemary leaves, minced

¾ cup quinoa, rinsed

¾ cup low-sodium vegetable broth

¾ cup unsweetened almond milk or regular milk

Sea salt

Juice of ½ orange

3 ounces Gruyère or sharp Cheddar cheese, shredded (1 packed cup)

Freshly ground black pepper

2 tablespoons snipped fresh chives

1. Preheat a small saucepan over medium-high heat.

2. When the saucepan is hot, drizzle in 1 tablespoon of oil, and add the shallots. Cook for 30 seconds, or until translucent and fragrant.

3. Add the mushrooms and rosemary. Sauté, stirring occasionally, for 3 to 4 minutes, or until the mushrooms start to brown.

4. Add the quinoa.

5. Reduce the heat to medium. Cook, stirring often, for about 4 minutes, or until the quinoa is lightly browned and smells nutty.

6. Stir in the broth, milk, and a pinch of salt. Bring to a boil.

7. Reduce the heat to maintain a simmer. Cover the pan, and cook for about 15 minutes, or until the quinoa is tender and the liquid has been absorbed. Remove from the heat.

8. Stir in the orange juice, remaining 1 tablespoon of oil, and the cheese until the cheese melts into the quinoa. Taste, and season with salt and pepper as needed.

9. Serve the porridge topped with the chives.

Beyond the basics: *To make the dish extra protein rich, add a poached egg on top.*

Per Serving: Calories: 305; Total fat: 18g; Carbohydrates: 25g; Fiber: 3g; Protein: 13g; Sodium: 200mg

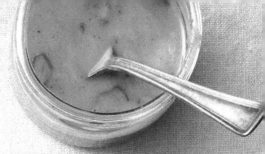

**Grilled Heirloom Tomatoes
with Spicy Tahini Dressing
Page 85**

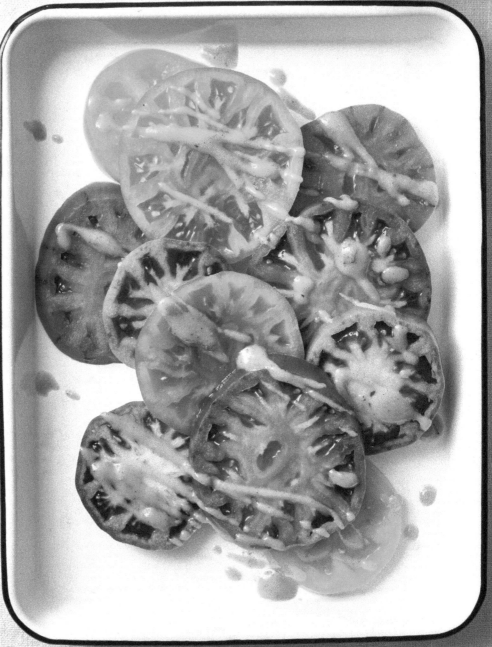

CHAPTER EIGHT

SNACKS + SMALL BITES

- - - - -

Grilled Salmon Bites with Dijon Mustard and Dill

SERVES 4 / ACTIVE TIME: 25 MINUTES

DAIRY-FREE, GLUTEN-FREE, NUT-FREE

This spring-like dish is the perfect bite of rich salmon, tangy Dijon mustard, and anise-like dill. Salmon is a great source of omega-3 fatty acids, and dill gives a boost of vitamin C. It's a simple dish that's big on protein and flavor.

3 tablespoons finely chopped fresh parsley

3 tablespoons olive oil

3 tablespoons freshly squeezed lemon juice

3 large garlic cloves, minced

2 tablespoons chopped fresh dill

1½ teaspoons Dijon mustard

1 teaspoon sea salt

½ teaspoon freshly ground black pepper

1½ pounds skinless salmon fillets, cut into 1-inch dice

1. Soak 8 small wooden skewers in water for at least 1 hour to keep them from catching fire on the grill.

2. Preheat a grill to 375°F.

3. To make the marinade, in a medium bowl, stir together the parsley, oil, lemon juice, garlic, dill, mustard, salt, and pepper. Divide between 2 medium bowls.

4. Toss the salmon in one bowl of marinade. Thread 2 or 3 salmon pieces onto each skewer.

5. Place the skewers on the hot grill. Grill for 3 to 4 minutes per side, or until the salmon is opaque. Remove from the heat. Serve hot, drizzled with the reserved marinade.

Make it easier: *Instead of grilling, cook the salmon skewers in a preheated sauté pan or skillet. They are less likely to break apart and fall into the grill.*

Per Serving: Calories: 349; Total fat: 22g; Carbohydrates: 4g; Fiber: 1g; Protein: 35g; Sodium: 505mg

Avocado, Hummus, and Chicken Quesadillas

SERVES 4 / ACTIVE TIME: 20 MINUTES

- -
DAIRY-FREE, GLUTEN-FREE, NUT-FREE
- -

We're dressing up our quesadillas in a slightly nontraditional way with homemade hummus, grilled chicken seasoned with ground cumin, and sliced avocado—they don't always have to include cheese. This recipe goes from snack to full meal with the addition of a salad and more vegetables.

1 pound boneless, skinless chicken breast

3 tablespoons olive oil, divided, plus more for grilling

1½ teaspoons ground cumin, divided

½ teaspoon garlic powder

Sea salt

Freshly ground black pepper

1 (15-ounce) can chickpeas, drained and rinsed

¼ cup tahini

1 garlic clove, peeled

Juice of ½ lemon

2 to 3 tablespoons water

1 ripe avocado

8 corn tortillas

1. Cut the chicken into long thin pieces. Transfer to a medium bowl.

2. Add 1 tablespoon of oil, ½ teaspoon of cumin, the garlic powder, and a pinch each of salt and pepper. Toss to coat.

3. Preheat a large skillet over medium-high heat.

4. When the skillet is hot, put the chicken in the skillet, and sauté, stirring occasionally, for 5 to 7 minutes, or until cooked through and no longer pink. Remove from the heat. Transfer the chicken to a plate.

5. To make the hummus, in a food processor, combine the chickpeas, tahini, garlic, lemon juice, 1 tablespoon of oil, the remaining 1 teaspoon of cumin, and a pinch each of salt and pepper. Blend until smooth and creamy.

6. Add the water to loosen the mixture and make it creamier.

7. Halve the avocado, remove the pit (see page 151), and using a spoon, scoop out the avocado meat. Cut into long thin slices.

8. Place 2 tortillas on a work surface. Spread each with the hummus.

>>

9. Sprinkle the chicken on 1 tortilla, and fan a few slices of avocado on top. Place the other tortilla on top, hummus-side down. Continue with the remaining tortillas and filling.

10. Preheat a large skillet over medium-high heat.

11. When the skillet is hot, reduce the heat to medium. Drizzle in the remaining 1 tablespoon of oil.

12. Working in batches of 1 to 3 quesadillas, place them in the skillet without overlapping. Grill for 4 to 5 minutes, or until the bottom is golden brown and looks crunchy.

13. Using a spatula, flip the quesadillas. Cook the other side for 3 to 4 minutes, or until golden brown and crispy. Remove from the heat. Quarter the quesadillas, and serve hot.

Healthy swap: *For a vegan quesadilla, replace the chicken with grilled portobello mushrooms, fresh tomato slices, or both.*

Per Serving: Calories: 584; Total fat: 31g; Carbohydrates: 45g; Fiber: 12g; Protein: 36g; Sodium: 260mg

Sweet Potato Fries with Homemade Ketchup

SERVES 4 / ACTIVE TIME: 15 MINUTES

DAIRY-FREE, GLUTEN-FREE, VEGETARIAN

A healthy-ish take on French fries, these sweet and savory fries are the perfect satisfying snack. The homemade ketchup features tomato paste, garlic, and spices without any strange additives or preservatives.

2 large sweet potatoes

3 recipes SPOOG (page 18), divided, plus more olive oil for drizzling

½ yellow onion, diced

2 teaspoons tomato paste

½ teaspoon ground mustard

½ teaspoon smoked paprika

Pinch ground cloves

Pinch ground allspice

¼ teaspoon red pepper flakes

1 (14½-ounce) can crushed tomatoes

2 tablespoons coconut sugar

2 tablespoons apple cider vinegar

1. Preheat the oven to 425°F. Line a baking sheet with parchment paper.

2. Rinse the sweet potatoes well, and cut them into long, thin slices. Transfer to a medium bowl.

3. Add 2 recipes of SPOOG, and toss to combine.

4. Spread the sweet potatoes out on the prepared baking sheet.

5. Transfer the baking sheet to the oven, and bake for 25 to 30 minutes, or until the sweet potatoes are tender and the edges are browning. Remove from the oven.

6. Preheat a small saucepan over medium heat.

7. Drizzle in a bit of oil, and add the onion. Sauté for 6 to 8 minutes, or until translucent, tender, and beginning to brown.

8. Stir in the tomato paste, remaining 1 recipe of SPOOG, the ground mustard, paprika, cloves, allspice, and red pepper flakes. Cook for about 1 minute, or until the tomato paste is evenly distributed and the spices are fragrant.

9. Stir in the tomatoes, sugar, and vinegar. Remove from the heat. Let cool. To make the ketchup, pour into a blender, and blend until smooth.

10. Serve the sweet potato fries with the ketchup on the side.

Beyond the basics: *Another vegetable that works well with sweet potato is parsnip. Prepare and bake the parsnips with the sweet potatoes, and serve with ketchup.*

Per Serving: Calories: 195; Total fat: 11g; Carbohydrates: 25g; Fiber: 5g; Protein: 2g; Sodium: 688mg

Grilled Heirloom Tomatoes with Spicy Tahini Dressing

SERVES 4 / ACTIVE TIME: 15 MINUTES

DAIRY-FREE, GLUTEN-FREE, NUT-FREE, VEGETARIAN

Heirloom tomatoes are like the gold medal of all tomatoes. Colorful and vibrant, oddly shaped, and delicious, these beauties brighten any dish. They are often open-pollinated by insects, birds, the wind, or other natural mechanisms. Dress them up with spicy tahini, and you've got the perfect end-of-summer tomato feast.

¼ cup tahini

¼ teaspoon cayenne pepper

Juice of ½ lemon

1 teaspoon Dijon mustard

6 large fresh basil leaves, thinly sliced

¼ cup extra-virgin olive oil, plus 1 tablespoon

Salt

Freshly ground black pepper

2 large heirloom tomatoes

1. Preheat a grill to 450°F.

2. In a small bowl, whisk together the tahini, cayenne, lemon juice, mustard, basil, ¼ cup of oil, and a pinch each of salt and pepper to blend.

3. Cut the tomatoes into thick steaks, 2 to 4 pieces each.

4. In a shallow bowl, toss the tomatoes with the remaining 1 tablespoon of oil and a pinch each of salt and pepper.

5. Put the tomatoes on the grill, and lightly grill for 1 to 2 minutes per side. Tomatoes are fragile, so be careful not to overgrill them. When finished, arrange them in a fan-like position on a plate, and drizzle with the sauce. Turn off the heat.

Make it easier: *The tomatoes don't need to be grilled if they are ripe and in season; they can be served fresh with the dressing.*

Per Serving: Calories: 257; Total fat: 25g; Carbohydrates: 7g; Fiber: 3g; Protein: 3g; Sodium: 75mg

Yogurt "Ranch" Dip

SERVES 2 / ACTIVE TIME: 15 MINUTES

GLUTEN-FREE, NUT-FREE, VEGETARIAN

This dip will make the whole family happy and take you back to childhood. This dip is much healthier than what's in the store. It has probiotic-rich yogurt that helps keep your tummy digesting properly, along with all sorts of nutrient-rich fresh herbs. Make a big batch to keep in the refrigerator all week for an easy snack with your favorite dippers, or toss with lettuce as a creamy salad dressing.

1 cup plain, full-fat Greek yogurt

1 tablespoon rice vinegar

2 teaspoons fresh dill, minced, or 1 teaspoon dried

2 teaspoons fresh chives, minced, or 1 teaspoon dried

2 teaspoons fresh parsley, minced, or 1 teaspoon dried

1 teaspoon garlic powder

1 teaspoon onion powder

½ teaspoon fine sea salt, plus more as needed

¼ teaspoon freshly ground black pepper, plus more as needed

In a small bowl, stir together the yogurt, vinegar, dill, chives, parsley, garlic powder, onion powder, salt, and pepper, or pulse together in a food processor. Taste, and season with more salt and pepper as needed. Cover, and refrigerate until ready to serve.

Make it healthier: *Instead of dipping chips in this "ranch" dip, dip carrots, celery, parsnips, and cucumbers for a light, refreshing, satisfying snack.*

Per Serving: Calories: 93; Total fat: 4g; Carbohydrates: 9g; Fiber: 1g; Protein: 5g; Sodium: 409mg

Prosciutto-Wrapped Dates Stuffed with Roasted Almonds

SERVES 4 / ACTIVE TIME: 10 MINUTES

DAIRY-FREE, GLUTEN-FREE

A perfect balance of salty and sweet, crunchy and soft, these bite-size treats are a luxurious snack or appetizer. You'll impress with these at your next dinner party.

8 almonds

8 medjool dates

2 ounces prosciutto, cut into 1-by-3-inch slices

1. Preheat the oven to 425°F.

2. Put the almonds on a small baking sheet.

3. Transfer the baking sheet to the oven, and roast for about 7 minutes, or until the almonds are toasted. Remove from the oven. Let cool.

4. Halve the dates on one side to remove and discard the pits. Stuff each date with 1 almond, and press the date together.

5. Wrap each date with the prosciutto—the prosciutto should stick to itself to seal. Serve at room temperature.

Beyond the basics: *To make this even more of a sweet and salty dish, drizzle honey over the prosciutto.*

Per Serving: Calories: 170; Total fat: 2g; Carbohydrates: 37g; Fiber: 4g; Protein: 4g; Sodium: 163mg

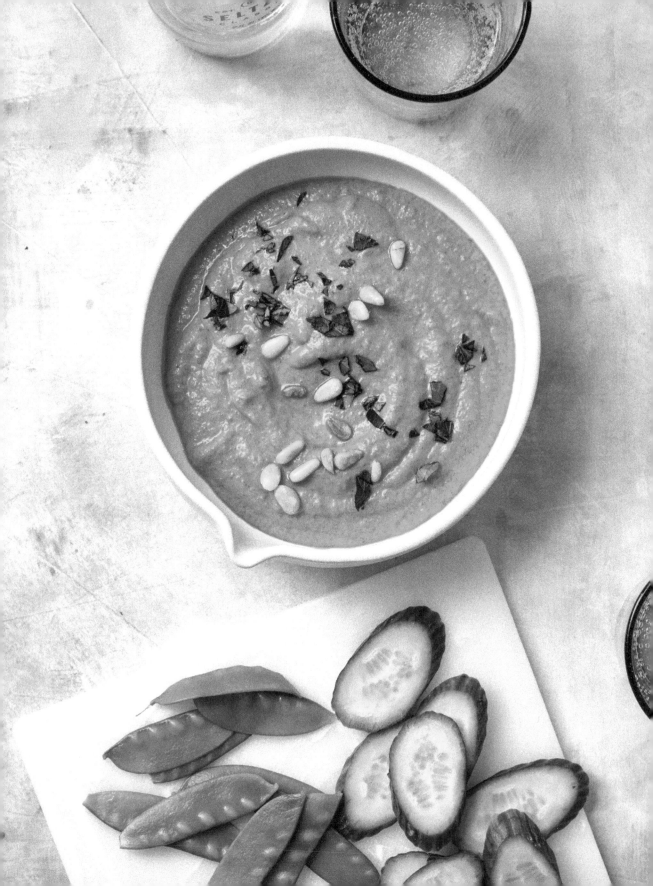

Beet Yogurt Dip with Cucumber "Chips"

SERVES 4 / ACTIVE TIME: 15 MINUTES

GLUTEN-FREE, NUT-FREE, VEGETARIAN

Beets are full of nutrients known to be detoxifying, help lower blood pressure, and improve heart health. The betalain pigment, which gives beets their rich color, is the source of many of these nutrients and vitamins. Of course, it also gives your food a fun, natural color.

FOR THE BEETS

2 large or 4 small red or orange beets

Grated zest of 1 orange

Juice of 1 orange

Pinch cayenne pepper

2 recipes SPOOG (page 18)

FOR THE DIP AND CUCUMBER

½ cup plain, full-fat Greek yogurt

1 garlic clove, peeled

Grated zest of ½ lemon

Juice of ½ lemon

1 teaspoon maple syrup

Pinch sea salt

Pinch cayenne pepper

1 tablespoon chopped fresh parsley (optional)

¼ cup pine nuts (optional)

1 large cucumber, cut into thin rounds

1. **To make the beets:** Preheat the oven to 425°F. Line a baking sheet with aluminum foil.

2. Rinse the beets, and place them in the middle of the foil.

3. Drizzle with the orange zest, orange juice, cayenne, and SPOOG. Bring up the sides of the foil, and wrap it around the beets. Tightly seal the foil, pinching it together at the top.

>>

4. Transfer the baking sheet to the oven, and bake for 40 to 50 minutes, or until the beets are tender. Remove from the oven. Let cool completely.

5. When cool enough to handle, remove the beets from the foil. Pour all the juices into a food processor. Using your fingers, peel off and discard the skins. Slice off any parts of the roots or pieces that don't look edible. Put the beets into the food processor.

6. **To make the dip and cucumber:** Add the yogurt, garlic, lemon zest, lemon juice, maple syrup, salt, and cayenne to the food processor. Process until smooth. Transfer to a bowl.

7. Garnish with the parsley and pine nuts (if using), and serve with the cucumber "chips" for dipping. The dip can also be served with additional crudités, if desired.

Beyond the basics: *Blend walnuts or pine nuts into the dip, or top it with chopped hazelnuts!*

Per Serving: Calories: 127; Total fat: 8g; Carbohydrates: 13g; Fiber: 2g; Protein: 2g; Sodium: 415mg

Frozen Almond Butter Yogurt Bites

SERVES 4 / ACTIVE TIME: 5 MINUTES

GLUTEN-FREE, VEGETARIAN

This is my version of frozen yogurt, whipped with creamy almond butter. These bites are a cold sweet treat that just so happens to be filled with protein and probiotics yet is light on sugar. A perfect go-to whenever you have a hankering for ice cream.

1½ cups plain, full-fat Greek yogurt

1 tablespoon maple syrup

¼ teaspoon sea salt

¼ cup unsalted almond butter

½ (4-ounce) 70 to 85 percent cocoa dark chocolate bar, chopped into chip-like pieces

1. In a medium bowl, whisk together the yogurt, maple syrup, and salt to blend.

2. Drizzle in the almond butter, and stir to swirl it into the yogurt.

3. Fill about 4 wells in a standard muffin tin with the yogurt mixture.

4. Sprinkle the chocolate pieces on top.

5. Insert 1 ice-pop stick into each muffin well. Freeze for 3 to 4 hours, or until solid.

Healthy swap: *Use honey instead of maple syrup. Honey is an antibacterial, and it is delicious.*

Per Serving: Calories: 244; Total fat: 16g; Carbohydrates: 19g; Fiber: 3g; Protein: 7g; Sodium: 161mg

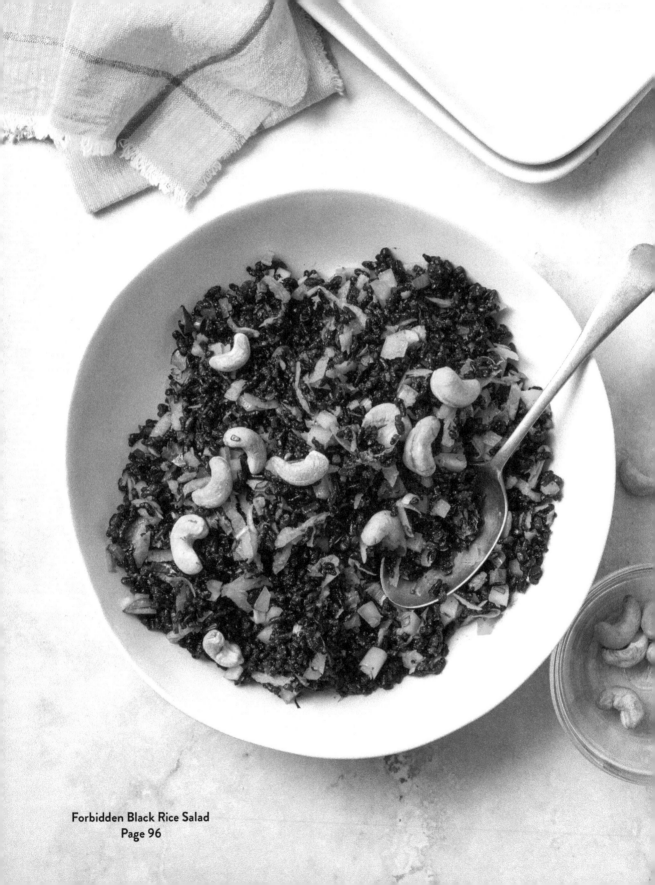

Forbidden Black Rice Salad
Page 96

CHAPTER NINE

SIGNED

Quinoa Risotto with Sautéed Asparagus and Sweet Peas

SERVES 4 / ACTIVE TIME: 30 MINUTES

GLUTEN-FREE, NUT-FREE, VEGETARIAN

If you want a flavor-packed, power-inducing meal, make this side dish! This recipe is so protein rich you could eat it as a main dish, especially with a poached egg on top. The asparagus is a liver detoxifier, and the sweet peas help control blood sugar.

2 leeks

1 bunch asparagus

3 tablespoons extra-virgin olive oil, divided

3 garlic cloves, minced

1 cup quinoa, rinsed

½ cup white wine

Juice of ½ lemon

Grated zest of ½ lemon

2 cups low-sodium vegetable broth

Sea salt

1 cup fresh or frozen peas

½ cup chopped fresh basil leaves

4 ounces pecorino or parmesan cheese, shaved

1. Thoroughly rinse the leeks under cold water, and pat dry using a towel. Using a sharp knife, cut off the dark, tough leaves at the part of the stalk where the color changes to light green. Discard the tough dark green leaves. Trim off the root end and discard. Cut the leeks into thin rounds, submerge in a bowl of cold water, and give them a stir to remove the grit between the layers. Using your hands or a slotted spoon, scoop the leeks out of the water, and drain in a colander.

2. Snap each asparagus spear at the natural breaking point, which is usually about halfway up. Discard the bottoms, which are not very edible. Cut the asparagus into large chunks.

3. Preheat a large pot over medium-high heat.

4. When the pot is hot, add 1 tablespoon of oil and the leeks. Cook for about 2 minutes, or until the leeks start to soften.

5. Add the asparagus. Cook, stirring occasionally, for 5 minutes, or until tender.

6. Stir in the garlic, and cook for about 1 minute to release their flavor.

7. Stir in the quinoa, wine, lemon juice, and lemon zest. Cook for 1 minute, or until the wine has been absorbed.

8. Add the broth. Season with salt. Cook, stirring often, for 15 minutes, or until the broth has been absorbed and the quinoa is puffed up and soft.

9. Add the peas. Cook, stirring, for about 3 minutes, or until the peas are soft and warm.

10. Stir in the basil, and cook for 1 minute. Turn off the heat.

11. Drizzle in the remaining 2 tablespoons of oil, and sprinkle on the cheese. Cover the pot, and let sit for about 2 minutes, or until the cheese is soft. Serve hot.

Healthy swap: *Skip the cheese, and add 2 tablespoons nutritional yeast plus ¼ cup pine nuts. This will give the quinoa a nutty, cheesy flavor, and you won't miss the cheese.*

Per Serving: Calories: 459; Total fat: 21g; Carbohydrates: 47g; Fiber: 7g; Protein: 18g; Sodium: 565mg

Forbidden Black Rice Salad

DAIRY-FREE, GLUTEN-FREE, VEGETARIAN

Forbidden black rice, because of its high levels of anthocyanin pigment, was forbidden to anyone but royalty in ancient China. This pigment is the same one that gives blackberries and eggplant their deep-purple color and supports heart, eye, and skin health. Compared to brown rice, and certainly white rice, black rice contains more protein and iron.

1 cup forbidden black rice or brown rice

2 cups water

½ red, yellow, or orange bell pepper, finely diced

½ large carrot, grated

1 scallion, green and white parts, chopped

½ cup chopped fresh cilantro

½ teaspoon sriracha or other chile sauce, plus more as needed

2 tablespoons sesame oil

1½ teaspoons garlic powder, plus more as needed

Grated zest of ½ lime

Juice of ½ lime

Sea salt

Freshly ground black pepper

¼ cup unsalted roasted cashews

1. In a medium pot, combine the rice and water. Cover the pot with a tight-fitting lid, and bring to a boil over high heat.

2. Reduce the heat to medium-low. Simmer the rice for about 40 minutes, or until the water has been absorbed and the rice is soft. Refrain from removing the lid while cooking to check the rice. Remove from the heat. Let the rice cool for 5 to 10 minutes.

3. Meanwhile, put the bell pepper, carrot, and scallion in a large serving bowl.

4. Add the cilantro, sriracha, oil, garlic powder, lime zest, and lime juice. Season with salt and pepper. Toss to combine.

5. Add the rice to the vegetables, and toss. Taste, and season with more salt, pepper, garlic powder, or sriracha as needed.

6. Sprinkle the cashews on top, and serve hot or cold.

Beyond the basics: *To make this into a vegetarian or vegan main dish, cook 1 cup dried lentils according to the package directions, and mix into the rice. Cut 1 ripe avocado into chunks, and sprinkle on top with the cashews.*

Per Serving: Calories: 298; Total fat: 12g; Carbohydrates: 43g; Fiber: 3g; Protein: 6g; Sodium: 51mg

Red Onion and Lentil Soup

SERVES 4 / ACTIVE TIME: 20 MINUTES

GLUTEN-FREE, NUT-FREE, VEGETARIAN

Lentils are one of my pantry staples. They are a wonderful option for a plant-based meal filled with protein, fiber, and delicious earthy flavor. They can be added to all types of soups and salads, either taking center stage or acting as a supporting ingredient.

¼ cup olive oil

2 red onions, halved, thinly cut into half-moons

3 garlic cloves, minced

3 bay leaves

5 thyme sprigs or 1 tablespoon dried thyme leaves

½ teaspoon sea salt, plus more as needed

¼ teaspoon freshly ground black pepper, plus more as needed

1 cup medium-bodied red wine, such as merlot or pinot noir

8 cups low-sodium vegetable broth

¾ cup dried black or green lentils

8 ounces Gruyère cheese, grated

1. Preheat a large pot over medium heat.

2. When the pot is hot, pour in the oil, and add the onions. Cook, stirring occasionally, for 2 to 3 minutes, or until translucent.

3. Add the garlic, bay leaves, thyme, salt, and pepper. Cook, stirring often, for 3 to 5 minutes, or until the onions are soft and tender.

4. Add the wine, and bring to a boil.

5. Add the broth and lentils. Return the soup to a boil.

6. Reduce the heat to medium to maintain a strong simmer. Cook for 10 to 15 minutes, or until the lentils are tender. Season with salt and pepper. Remove from the heat. Discard the bay leaves.

7. Ladle the soup into bowls, sprinkle the cheese on top, and let sit for 1 minute to let melt slightly.

Healthy swap: *To avoid alcohol, substitute 2 tablespoons apple cider vinegar for the wine.*

Per Serving: Calories: 552; Total fat: 30g; Carbohydrates: 39g; Fiber: 5g; Protein: 25g; Sodium: 863mg

Sweet Pea, Goat Cheese, and Avocado Salad with Lemon Vinaigrette

SERVES 4 / ACTIVE TIME: 15 MINUTES

GLUTEN-FREE, VEGETARIAN

This springtime salad is a beautiful green, citrusy, salty medley of butter lettuce, sweet peas, and creamy avocado with plenty of different textures in each bite.

1 cup pine nuts

2 ripe avocados

4 cups coarsely torn butter lettuce or little gem lettuce leaves (about 2 bunches)

4 ounces sugar snap peas, trimmed, thinly sliced (about 1 cup)

Grated zest of 1 lemon

Juice of 1 lemon, plus more as needed

4 recipes SPOOG (page 18), plus more salt and pepper as needed

2 tablespoons honey, plus more as needed

2 tablespoons white-wine vinegar

1 teaspoon Dijon mustard

4 ounces goat cheese, crumbled

1. Preheat the oven to 400°F.

2. Spread the pine nuts out on a baking sheet.

3. Transfer the baking sheet to the oven, and roast for 5 minutes, watching closely so the pine nuts don't burn. Remove from the oven.

4. Halve the avocados, remove the pits (see page 151), and using a spoon, scoop out the avocado meat. Cut into large chunks.

5. In a large salad bowl, combine the lettuce, avocados, and sugar snap peas.

6. In a small saucepan, combine the lemon zest, lemon juice, SPOOG, and honey. Bring to a light simmer over low heat. Cook, stirring occasionally, for about 3 minutes. Remove from the heat. Let cool for a couple of minutes, then transfer to a blender.

7. Add the vinegar and mustard. Blend well. Taste, and season with more lemon juice, honey, salt, and pepper if needed.

8. Top the salad with the pine nuts and cheese. Drizzle with the dressing to serve.

Per Serving: Calories: 665; Total fat: 59g; Carbohydrates: 31g; Fiber: 11g; Protein: 15g; Sodium: 799mg

Roasted Butternut Squash with Cranberries and Caramelized Onion

SERVES 4 / ACTIVE TIME: 20 MINUTES

DAIRY-FREE, GLUTEN-FREE, NUT-FREE, VEGETARIAN

Butternut squash is full of sweetness and nutty flavor. Tart cranberries and tender, sweet onion add an exquisite complement that makes for a great addition to my Rosemary Lamb Chops (page 52).

1 butternut squash, peeled, seeded, and cut into ½-inch dice

3 tablespoons olive oil, divided

¾ teaspoon sea salt, divided

½ teaspoon freshly ground black pepper, plus a pinch

3 garlic cloves, minced, divided, or 1 teaspoon dried granulated garlic

½ yellow onion, cut into ½-inch dice

2 tablespoons minced fresh sage leaves

½ cup unsweetened dried cranberries, coarsely chopped

1. Preheat the oven to 425°F. Line 2 baking sheets with parchment paper.

2. In a large bowl, combine the squash, 2 tablespoons of oil, ½ teaspoon of salt, the pepper, and half of the garlic. Toss to combine.

3. Spread the squash out on one of the prepared baking sheets so the squash pieces do not overlap.

4. Transfer the baking sheet to the oven, and roast for 30 to 40 minutes, or until the squash is brown on the outside and very tender (do not undercook the squash). Remove from the oven.

5. While the squash roasts, on the remaining prepared baking sheet, toss together the onion, remaining 1 tablespoon of oil, remaining ¼ teaspoon of salt, pinch of pepper, and the remaining garlic.

6. Transfer the baking sheet to the oven, and roast for 20 minutes, or until the onion is lightly browned, tender, and slightly caramelized. Remove from the oven.

7. In a large bowl, toss together the squash, onion, sage, and cranberries. Serve hot or at room temperature.

Per Serving: Calories: 224; Total fat: 11g; Carbohydrates: 35g; Fiber: 5g; Protein: 2g; Sodium: 299mg

Roasted Parsnips with Roasted Red Pepper–Walnut Sauce

SERVES 4 / ACTIVE TIME: 15 MINUTES

DAIRY-FREE, GLUTEN-FREE, VEGETARIAN

A simple and healthier version of fries that tastes like candy. If you can't find parsnips, use sweet potatoes instead.

1 cup walnuts

2 pounds parsnips, cut into long, thin sticks

2 recipes SPOOG (page 18)

2 tablespoons olive oil

3 garlic cloves, minced

1 jarred roasted red pepper, drained

2 tablespoons water

1½ tablespoons tomato paste

1½ tablespoons sherry vinegar

1 teaspoon smoked paprika

½ teaspoon sea salt

¼ teaspoon chili powder

1. Preheat the oven to 425°F. Line a baking sheet with parchment paper.

2. Spread the walnuts out on an unlined baking sheet.

3. Transfer the baking sheet to the oven, and toast for 5 to 7 minutes, or until the walnuts start to brown and are fragrant, watching closely so they don't burn. Remove from the oven.

4. In a large bowl, toss together the parsnips and SPOOG.

5. Spread the parsnips out on the prepared baking sheet.

6. Transfer the baking sheet to the oven, and roast for 15 to 20 minutes, or until the parsnips are tender. Remove from the oven.

7. Preheat a small skillet over medium heat for 30 to 60 seconds, or until warm.

8. Pour in the oil, and add the garlic. Sauté for 2 minutes, or until fragrant, soft, and slightly brown. Do not cook the garlic until it is dark brown; at that point it is burnt and too late. Remove from the heat. Transfer to a food processor.

9. To make the sauce, add the roasted red pepper, walnuts, water, tomato paste, vinegar, paprika, salt, and chili powder. Blend until smooth.

10. Serve the sauce drizzled over the roasted parsnips or as a dip.

Per Serving: Calories: 500; Total fat: 34g; Carbohydrates: 49g; Fiber: 14g; Protein: 8g; Sodium: 644mg

Eggplant Strips with Cocoa, Garlic, Pine Nuts, and Basil Yogurt

SERVES 4 / ACTIVE TIME: 15 MINUTES

GLUTEN-FREE, VEGETARIAN

This roasted eggplant has an irresistible smoky flavor, complemented by sweet and earthy cocoa, sharp and spicy garlic, buttery pine nuts, and tangy yogurt. This is a great side for most Mediterranean-inspired dishes.

¼ cup pine nuts

3 medium eggplants, trimmed

¼ cup olive oil, plus 2 tablespoons, divided

1¼ teaspoons sea salt, divided

Pinch freshly ground black pepper

2 garlic cloves, peeled

2 tablespoons freshly squeezed lemon juice

1 teaspoon molasses or maple syrup

1 teaspoon cocoa powder

½ teaspoon chili powder

⅓ cup plain, full-fat Greek yogurt

½ cup fresh basil leaves, chopped

1. Preheat the oven to 400°F.

2. Spread the pine nuts out on a baking sheet.

3. Transfer the baking sheet to the oven, and roast for 5 minutes, watching closely so the pine nuts don't burn. Remove from the oven.

4. Increase the oven temperature to 425°F. Line a baking sheet with parchment paper.

5. Halve the eggplants lengthwise, then again crosswise. Cut each section into strips about 1 inch thick and 4 inches long. Transfer to a large bowl.

6. Add ¼ cup of oil, 1 teaspoon of salt, and the pepper. Mix well.

7. Spread the eggplants onto the prepared baking sheet so the pieces are not crowded.

8. Transfer the baking sheet to the oven, and roast for about 40 minutes, or until the eggplants are golden brown on the outside and tender. It is important not to undercook the eggplants, since they will not taste good. Remove from the oven. Let cool.

9. In a food processor, combine the remaining 2 tablespoons of oil, the garlic, lemon juice, molasses, cocoa powder, chili powder, and remaining ¼ teaspoon of salt. Process for about 2 minutes, or until smooth.

10. Scoop the yogurt onto a serving plate, and spread it out slightly.

11. Arrange the roasted eggplant on top, and drizzle with the molasses mixture.

12. Sprinkle with the basil and pine nuts. Serve at room temperature.

Beyond the basics: *If you make this ahead, toss the eggplant into the molasses mixture, and let it marinate for a few hours. The flavors will create a big bang.*

Per Serving: Calories: 362; Total fat: 28g; Carbohydrates: 29g; Fiber: 13g; Protein: 6g; Sodium: 68mg

Sherry-Braised Green Beans

SERVES 4 / ACTIVE TIME: 20 MINUTES

DAIRY-FREE, GLUTEN-FREE, NUT-FREE, VEGETARIAN

Sherry adds a hint of acidity to these bright, tender, low-calorie green beans. Garlic adds dynamic flavor and is also great for fighting off colds and supporting the immune system. I recommend enjoying these beans with my Lamb Steak and Roasted Vegetables (page 128). If you cannot find sherry, you can use sherry vinegar as an alternative, but cut the amount in half.

2 leeks

1 tablespoon olive oil

2 pounds green beans, trimmed and halved

4 garlic cloves, minced

¼ cup sherry or white wine

Grated zest of 1 lemon

Juice of 1 lemon

1. Thoroughly rinse the leeks under cold water, and pat dry using a towel. Using a sharp knife, cut off the dark, tough leaves at the part of the stalk where the color changes to light green. Discard the tough dark green leaves. Trim off the root end and discard. Cut the leeks into thin rounds, submerge in a bowl of cold water, and give them a stir to remove the grit between the layers. Using your hands or a slotted spoon, scoop the leeks out of the water, and drain in a colander.

2. Preheat a large skillet over medium-high heat.

3. Drizzle in the oil, and add the leeks. Cook, stirring halfway through, for about 1 minute, or until fragrant and slightly translucent.

4. Add the green beans, and cook for 4 to 5 minutes without interruption, or until browned nicely on the first side.

5. Add the garlic, stir, and cook for 1 to 2 minutes, or until fragrant and the flavors have melded.

6. Once the green beans have browned on both sides, add the sherry, lemon zest, and lemon juice. Shake the skillet, and let the liquid come to a simmer.

7. Reduce the heat to medium-low. Cover the skillet, and cook the beans for 8 to 10 minutes, or until most of the liquid has been absorbed and the beans are tender. Remove from the heat. Serve hot.

Per Serving: Calories: 146; Total fat: 4g; Carbohydrates: 24g; Fiber: 7g; Protein: 5g; Sodium: 24mg

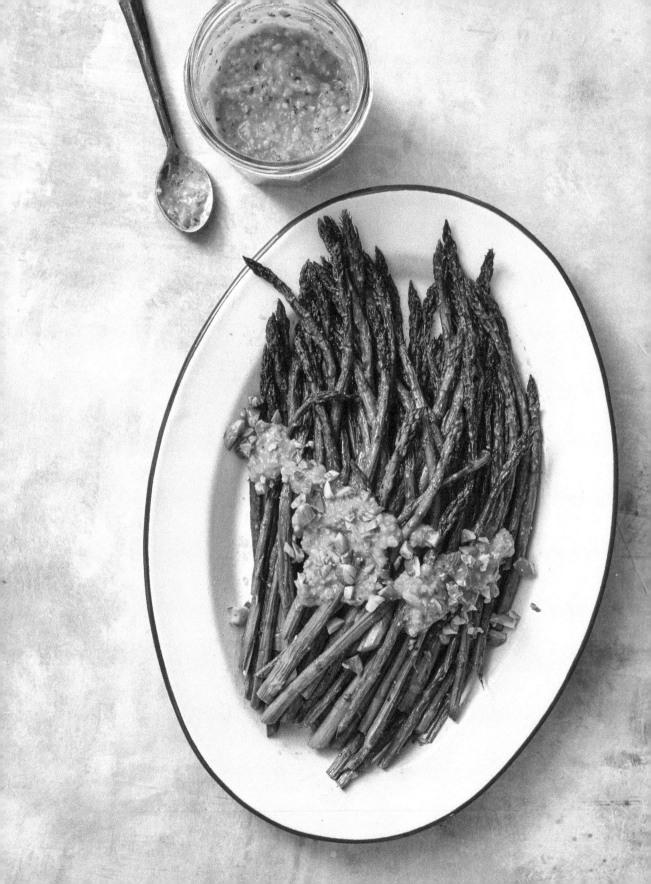

Roasted Asparagus with Romesco Sauce

SERVES 4 / ACTIVE TIME: 15 MINUTES

DAIRY-FREE, GLUTEN-FREE, VEGETARIAN

Salt, pepper, olive oil, and garlic powder are practically all you need to make any vegetable or meat taste delicious, including asparagus. But this romesco sauce, with origins from Spain, adds a smoky rich flavor brimming with tomatoes, roasted red pepper, garlic, and toasted almonds.

FOR THE ASPARAGUS

2 pounds thin asparagus

2 recipes SPOOG (page 18)

FOR THE ROMESCO SAUCE

½ cup almonds

½ cup extra-virgin olive oil

1 jarred roasted red pepper

¼ cup tomato puree

2 garlic cloves, peeled

2 tablespoons chopped fresh flat-leaf parsley

3 tablespoons freshly squeezed lemon juice

1 teaspoon smoked paprika

Pinch sea salt, plus more as needed

Pinch freshly ground black pepper, plus more as needed

2 tablespoons sliced almonds

1. **To make the asparagus:** Preheat the oven to 425°F. Line two baking sheets with parchment paper.

2. Snap each asparagus spear at the natural breaking point, which is usually about halfway up. Discard the bottoms, which are not very edible.

3. In a medium bowl, toss together the asparagus and SPOOG.

4. Spread the asparagus out on the prepared baking sheets.

5. Transfer the baking sheets to the oven—one on the lower rack and one on the upper rack—and roast for 5 to 8 minutes, or until the asparagus is golden brown on the outside and tender. Remove from the oven, leaving the oven on.

6. **To make the romesco sauce:** Reduce the oven temperature to 400°F.

7. Spread the almonds out on a baking sheet.

8. Transfer to the oven, and toast for 7 minutes, or until the almonds are browned and fragrant, watching closely so they don't burn. Remove from the oven. Let cool.

>>

9. In a food processor, combine the toasted almonds, oil, roasted red pepper, tomato puree, garlic, parsley, lemon juice, paprika, salt, and pepper. Pulse until thick and slightly chunky. Taste, and season with more salt and pepper if needed.

10. Serve the hot asparagus with the romesco sauce on top. Garnish with the sliced almonds.

Beyond the basics: *If you want to make a thinner sauce, add 2 tablespoons water, and puree the sauce longer. This will be nice for plating a fancier dinner.*

Per Serving: Calories: 402; Total fat: 38g; Carbohydrates: 15g; Fiber: 7g; Protein: 8g; Sodium: 339mg

Spinach Salad with Cider Vinegar, Honey, and Olive Oil Drizzle

SERVES 4 / ACTIVE TIME: 25 MINUTES

DAIRY-FREE, GLUTEN-FREE, VEGETARIAN

A warming, wintery dish that is still fresh, light, and healthy. This veggie-full salad will satisfy your craving for something abundant in nutrients, quick, and tasty. It is a delicious combination of savory, sweet, citrus, and nutty. Keep an eye on the nuts while they bake—they burn quickly.

1 pound fresh baby spinach

1 pound broccoli, cut into bite-size chunks

2 teaspoons extra-virgin olive oil, plus 2 tablespoons, divided

Sea salt

Freshly ground black pepper

1 cup pecans

1 teaspoon ground cinnamon

Pinch cayenne pepper

2 oranges

1 tablespoon apple cider vinegar

1 tablespoon honey

1. Preheat the oven to 400°F.

2. Rinse the spinach, and let sit in open air on a towel to dry well.

3. Set a steamer basket in a large pot, and fill the pot with ½ inch of water, making sure the water does not touch the basket. Bring to a boil.

4. Add the broccoli to the steamer basket, cover the pot, and steam for about 5 minutes, or just until tender. Remove from the heat. Transfer to a large serving bowl.

5. Add 1 teaspoon of oil and a pinch each of salt and pepper. Toss to combine.

6. In a small bowl, toss together the pecans, 1 teaspoon of oil, the cinnamon, cayenne, and a pinch each of salt and pepper.

7. Spread the pecans out on a baking sheet.

8. Transfer the baking sheet to the oven, and bake for about 7 minutes, or until the pecans are toasted but not burnt. Remove from the oven. Let cool.

>>

9. Using a sharp knife, trim off the skin and outside white layer of pith from the oranges so the juicy flesh is exposed. One at a time, holding the orange in your palm over a small bowl to catch the juice, press the whole edge of the knife into the orange between the white membranes to separate the orange segments from the membrane. Put the segments in another small bowl. Squeeze any remaining juice from the membranes into the first bowl, and discard the membranes.

10. In another small bowl, whisk together the vinegar, honey, 1 tablespoon of orange juice from segmenting the oranges, a pinch of salt, and a couple good cranks of pepper until well combined.

11. While whisking, slowly pour in the remaining 2 tablespoons of oil to emulsify the vinaigrette.

12. Add the spinach, pecans, and orange segments to the bowl with the broccoli. Toss with some, or all, of the vinaigrette, as you like. Serve immediately.

Beyond the basics: *Nuts are a fun, nutritious addition to salads, and you can prep candied and spiced nuts in bulk and keep them in a jar until needed. If you want candied pecans here, toss them in 2 tablespoons maple syrup before putting into the oven on a baking sheet lined with parchment paper (so they don't stick to the pan). Let cool completely before using so the sugar hardens and becomes crunchy.*

Per Serving: Calories: 383; Total fat: 30g; Carbohydrates: 28g; Fiber: 10g; Protein: 9g; Sodium: 166mg

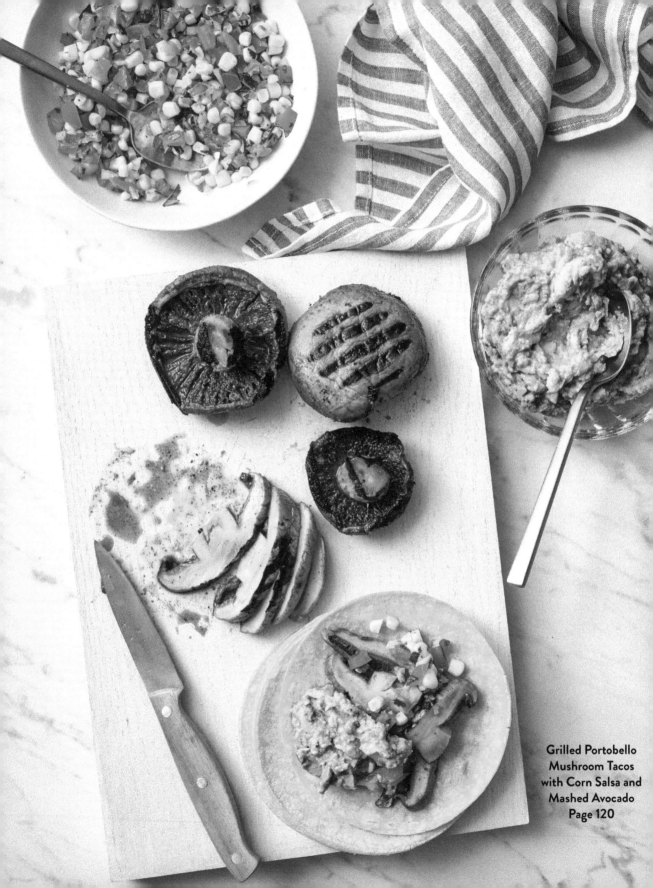

Grilled Portobello
Mushroom Tacos
with Corn Salsa and
Mashed Avocado
Page 120

CHAPTER TEN

MAIN DISHES

- - - - -

Socca with Caramelized Onion and Shiitake Mushroom

SERVES 4 / ACTIVE TIME: 20 MINUTES

GLUTEN-FREE, NUT-FREE, VEGETARIAN

Socca, also known as farinata, is believed to have originated in Genoa, Italy, making its way along the Mediterranean coast to southern France where it gained great popularity. This chickpea flour flatbread is versatile and the perfect vehicle for an assortment of sautéed veggies, spices, and cheeses.

1 cup chickpea flour

¾ teaspoon fine sea salt, plus more for seasoning

½ teaspoon freshly ground black pepper, plus more for seasoning

1¼ cups warm water

3 tablespoons olive oil, plus more for the skillet

1 large yellow or red onion, diced

1 pound shiitake mushrooms, quartered

½ teaspoon garlic powder

1 bunch fresh dill, coarsely chopped (optional)

8 ounces feta cheese, crumbled (optional)

1. In a large bowl, whisk together the flour, salt, pepper, water, and oil to combine. Cover the bowl, and let sit at room temperature for at least 30 minutes, but preferably 8 to 10 hours.

2. Preheat a large skillet over medium-high heat.

3. When the skillet is hot, reduce the heat to medium. Using a paper towel, carefully rub a bit of oil all over the skillet.

4. Pour in about one-fourth of the chickpea batter, and tilt the skillet so it coats the bottom evenly (it should resemble a large tortilla). Cook for 5 to 8 minutes, or until bubbles form on the surface and the batter turns from shiny to opaque.

5. Carefully flip the socca, and cook for 2 to 3 minutes, or until it browns slightly. Transfer to a plate, and cover with a towel to keep warm, or keep in an oven preheated to 200°F. Repeat with the remaining batter.

6. Reduce the heat to medium. Drizzle in more oil.

7. Add the onion, and cook for about 1 minute, or until it starts to turn translucent.

8. Add the mushrooms and garlic powder. Give it a quick stir, and cook, stirring often, for 7 to 8 minutes, or until the mushrooms are seared on the outside and tender inside. Remove from the heat. Transfer to a plate. Cover to keep warm.

9. Top each socca with the mushrooms, onion, a pinch of fresh dill (if using), and cheese (if using). Fold in half, and serve hot.

Beyond the basics: *Make these heartier with more protein-rich vegetables in the sauté, such as diced eggplant, fresh spinach, and diced bell pepper. Another cheese that would be tasty instead of feta would be 8 ounces crumbled goat cheese or 8 ounces grated Gruyère.*

Per Serving: Calories: 233; Total fat: 12g; Carbohydrates: 25g; Fiber: 6g; Protein: 8g; Sodium: 318mg

Spelt Margherita Calzones

SERVES 4 / ACTIVE TIME: 20 MINUTES

NUT-FREE, VEGETARIAN

Spelt is an ancient grain very closely related to wheat (so it is not gluten-free). Whole grains like spelt contain a fair amount of good carbs, protein, and fiber. They make for a delicious, hearty calzone, filled with juicy tomatoes and gooey mozzarella cheese.

3½ cups whole spelt flour, plus more as needed

1 teaspoon fine sea salt, divided

3 tablespoons extra-virgin olive oil, divided

1½ tablespoons active dry yeast

1 cup lukewarm water, plus more as needed

½ cup canned low-sodium pureed tomatoes

1 tablespoon balsamic vinegar

1 teaspoon dried oregano

½ teaspoon garlic powder

¼ to 1 teaspoon red pepper flakes (depending on desired heat level)

1 (8-ounce) ball mozzarella cheese, cut into thin rounds

4 ounces parmesan cheese, grated

1 bunch fresh basil leaves, cut into thin ribbons

1. Sift the flour into a large bowl.

2. Whisk in ½ teaspoon of salt and 2 tablespoons of oil to combine.

3. In a medium bowl, dissolve the yeast in the water.

4. Using one hand, little by little, stir the yeast water into the flour. If still very dry, drizzle in a little more water. If very wet, sprinkle in a little more flour. The dough should be moist but not wet and sticky.

5. Knead the dough by pressing your palm on it and folding it over for about 30 seconds, or until smooth. Be careful not to overwork the dough because that will result in tough and chewy calzones. You will know it is overworked if it loses its elasticity.

6. Shape the dough into a ball, then lightly dust with flour. Cover with a slightly damp towel, and allow to rest for 2 hours at room temperature, or until doubled in size.

7. About 10 minutes before forming the calzones, set an oven rack in the bottom position, and preheat the oven to 550°F. Line 2 baking sheets with parchment paper.

8. In a medium bowl, mix together the tomatoes, vinegar, oregano, garlic powder, remaining ½ teaspoon of salt, and the red pepper flakes.

9. Divide the spelt dough into 4 balls. Dust a work surface with flour, and roll each ball into a 10-inch round on it.

10. Place the dough rounds on the prepared baking sheets. Over half of each round, spread the tomato sauce.

11. Top the sauce with the mozzarella cheese, parmesan cheese, and a pinch of fresh basil. Fold the other half of the dough over, and pinch the edges together, making sure the dough is sealed.

12. Transfer the baking sheets to the bottom rack of the oven, and bake for 8 to 12 minutes, or until the calzones are golden. Remove from the oven.

13. Drizzle the calzones with the remaining 1 tablespoon of oil, and sprinkle more basil on top. Serve hot.

Make it easier: *If you can't find spelt flour, replace it with whole-wheat flour or all-purpose flour.*

Per Serving: Calories: 762; Total fat: 34g; Carbohydrates: 85g; Fiber: 13g; Protein: 37g; Sodium: 983mg

Thai-Inspired Coconut and Sweet Potato Soup

SERVES 4 / ACTIVE TIME: 20 MINUTES

DAIRY-FREE, GLUTEN-FREE, VEGETARIAN

This nourishing soup is filling and satisfying with just vegetables. Coconut milk is a wonderful source of healthy fat and a great way to make a dish creamy and thick without the use of dairy cream. Sweet potatoes are rich in vitamins, potassium, and fiber. The vegetables absorb the broth, creating a rich, comforting soup.

1 tablespoon coconut oil

1 teaspoon minced peeled fresh ginger

2 tablespoons green curry paste

2 large sweet potatoes, diced

4 cups full-fat coconut milk

4 cups low-sodium vegetable broth

2 bay leaves

Sea salt

1 lime, halved, plus more as needed

1 large bell pepper, seeded and cut into 1-inch dice

1 (15-ounce) can chickpeas, drained and rinsed

1 bunch fresh cilantro, coarsely chopped

1. Preheat a large pot or Dutch oven over medium-high heat.

2. When the pot is hot, pour in the oil to melt.

3. Stir in the ginger and curry paste. Sauté for 1 minute to activate the flavors.

4. Stir in the sweet potatoes.

5. Reduce the heat to medium. Cook, stirring occasionally, for 4 to 5 minutes to start the cooking process.

6. Stir in the coconut milk, broth, and bay leaves, making sure no vegetables are stuck to the bottom of the pot.

7. Increase the heat to high. Bring the liquid to a boil.

8. Reduce the heat to maintain a high simmer, and cook for 10 minutes, or until the sweet potatoes start softening but are still firm. Season with salt.

9. Stir in the juice of ½ lime, the bell pepper, and chickpeas. Cook for 10 minutes, or until the vegetables have softened and the sweet potatoes are extra tender.

10. Add three-fourths of the cilantro. Cook, stirring often, until the cilantro wilts into the soup. Taste the soup one more time, and add salt and more lime juice if needed. Remove from the heat and discard the bay leaves.

11. Serve the soup hot, topped with the remaining cilantro. If you have any lime left, quarter it for garnish.

Beyond the basics: *All sorts of vegetables can be added to this dish, including zucchini, Swiss chard, mushrooms, and pumpkin. You can also add sliced cooked chicken.*

Per Serving: Calories: 635; Total fat: 54g; Carbohydrates: 38g; Fiber: 8g; Protein: 11g; Sodium: 229mg

White Bean "Fondue" with Steamed Brussels Sprouts and Carrot Dippers

SERVES 4 / ACTIVE TIME: 20 MINUTES

DAIRY-FREE, NUT-FREE, VEGETARIAN

I crave those dark, cold, winter nights getting comfortable in a local restaurant and digging into their specialty: fondue. I could eat this every night. But in reality, all that cheese and wine is a lot for the gut to handle. Here is a lighter, healthier version for when you're craving fondue but don't need all that cheese. Beans are an incredible source of protein, in place of meat or other protein sources. They also pair perfectly with roasted Brussels sprouts, which are rich in antioxidants and omega-3 fatty acids.

2 pounds Brussels sprouts, trimmed and halved lengthwise

2 pounds carrots, cut into 2-inch-thick rounds

2½ recipes SPOOG (page 18), divided

3 cups unsalted canned white beans, drained and rinsed

½ cup tahini

½ cup nutritional yeast or finely grated Gruyère cheese

4 garlic cloves, peeled

2 tablespoons liquid aminos or low-sodium soy sauce

1 teaspoon freshly squeezed lemon juice

1 teaspoon Dijon mustard

1 teaspoon honey or maple syrup

1 whole-grain unsliced bread loaf, cut into thick cubes

1. Set a steamer basket in a large pot, and fill the pot with salted water, making sure the water reaches just below the basket. Bring to a boil.

2. Put the Brussels sprouts and carrots in the basket. Cover the pot with a lid, and steam for about 8 minutes, or until the vegetables are tender. Remove from the heat. Discard the water, and return the vegetables to the pot.

3. Add 2 recipes of SPOOG, toss to coat, and cover to keep warm.

4. In a blender, combine the beans, tahini, nutritional yeast, garlic, remaining ½ recipe of SPOOG, the liquid aminos, lemon juice, mustard, and honey. Blend on high speed, adding up to 1½ cups of water if needed to loosen the mixture and make it smooth and creamy. It should be a thick, cheese-like sauce.

5. Pour the blended mixture into a fondue pot or large saucepan that you can place on a table. Heat over medium heat just until the fondue starts to bubble. Remove from the heat.

6. Serve the fondue immediately with the steamed vegetables and fresh bread as dippers.

Healthy swap: *For a gluten-free option, substitute 2 pounds Yukon Gold potatoes, cubed, for the bread. Preheat the oven to 425°F. Toss the potatoes in 1 recipe SPOOG, and transfer to a baking sheet. Roast for 20 to 30 minutes, or until browned and tender.*

Per Serving: Calories: 999; Total fat: 36g; Carbohydrates: 135g; Fiber: 41g; Protein: 45g; Sodium: 1,437mg

Grilled Portobello Mushroom Tacos with Corn Salsa and Mashed Avocado

SERVES 4 / ACTIVE TIME: 25 MINUTES

GLUTEN-FREE, NUT-FREE, VEGETARIAN

My family LOVES Mexican food, whether in Mexico, in California, or at home. Portobello mushrooms have a meaty, thick texture and earthy flavor, making them a great substitute for meats. Not to mention, they're delicious and versatile and contain beneficial minerals and vitamins. They are the perfect centerpiece for these tacos, adorned with creamy avocado and corn salsa.

4 large portobello mushrooms

2 tablespoons liquid aminos

3 recipes SPOOG (page 18), divided

Juice of 3 limes, divided

2 teaspoons gluten-free Mexican-style seasoning blend

2 ears corn, kernels cut from the cob, or 1 cup frozen corn kernels

2 roma tomatoes, diced

½ red onion, finely diced

¼ to 1 serrano chile (depending on how spicy you like it; ¼ being mild, 1 being very hot), seeded and minced

½ bunch fresh cilantro, chopped

8 corn tortillas

2 ripe avocados

1. In a sealed container, combine the mushrooms, liquid aminos, 2 recipes of SPOOG, the juice of 1 lime, and the Mexican-style seasoning. Let sit at room temperature for 30 minutes, or refrigerate for up to 8 hours. The more time, the more flavor.

2. To make the salsa, in a medium bowl, stir together the corn, tomatoes, onion, serrano chile, cilantro, and juice of 1½ limes. Add half of the remaining SPOOG. Taste, and add more if needed. Cover, and refrigerate until needed. The flavors come together even better with time.

3. Preheat a grill between 450°F and 500°F.

4. When the grill is hot, put the mushrooms on the grill, and cook for about 5 minutes, or until dark grill marks appear.

5. Flip the mushrooms, and grill the other side for about 5 minutes, or until grill marks appear. Remove from the heat. Cover with aluminum foil, and let sit for about 5 minutes to absorb the juices.

6. Using a chef's knife, cut the mushrooms into long thin strips. Reserve under foil to keep warm.

7. Wrap the tortillas in foil, and put on the grill for 1 to 2 minutes, or until the tortillas are warmed and softened.

8. Halve the avocados, remove the pits (see page 151), and using a spoon, scoop the avocado meat into a bowl.

9. Add the remaining SPOOG and a squeeze of lime juice. Using a fork, mash the avocado to incorporate the flavors. Taste, and adjust the seasoning to your liking.

10. To compose the tacos, place a warm tortilla on a work surface. Fill it with the sliced mushrooms (about ½ mushroom per tortilla), and top with the corn salsa and avocado mash. Repeat for the remaining tacos, then eat immediately.

Beyond the basics: *For more "meat" in these tacos, sauté some plant-based ground beef with similar flavors as the mushroom marinade. It will add a delicious, hearty, healthy layer to the tacos. If you want to add something cold and refreshing to the taco, add a scoop of plain Greek yogurt.*

Per Serving: Calories: 464; Total fat: 29g; Carbohydrates: 52g; Fiber: 15g; Protein: 11g; Sodium: 824mg

Poached Lemon-Thyme Scallops with Fingerling Potatoes

SERVES 4 / ACTIVE TIME: 30 MINUTES

DAIRY-FREE, GLUTEN-FREE, NUT-FREE

When I think of scallops, I think of my sister Kelsey (because they are her favorite!), and I think of my Host Mom in France, Sylvie, who loved to make St. Jacques (scallops) poached in wine and butter. Poaching is a great way to cook cleanly, and here we are making a healthier version of Sylvie's St. Jacques. Fingerling potatoes make me think of France, too—they serve them with almost everything, cooked to perfection. I recommend adding a vegetable to these, such as Sherry-Braised Green Beans (page 103).

2 pounds fingerling potatoes

Sea salt

4 tablespoons olive oil, divided, plus more for drizzling

2 shallots, minced

2 pounds scallops

Grated zest of 2 lemons

Juice of 2 lemons, divided

4 thyme sprigs, divided

½ cup chopped fresh flat-leaf parsley, plus pinch

Freshly ground black pepper

2 cups water

1. Put the potatoes in a large pot of salted water. Bring to a boil.

2. Reduce the heat to maintain a low simmer. Cook for about 10 minutes, or until the potatoes are tender when pierced with a fork. Remove from the heat. Drain.

3. While the potatoes cook, preheat a deep skillet over medium-high heat.

4. When the skillet is hot, reduce the heat to medium. Pour in 2 tablespoons of oil, and add the shallots. Cook, stirring occasionally, for 1 to 2 minutes, or until the shallots begin to turn translucent.

5. Add the scallops, and sear for about 3 to 4 minutes, or until browned on the bottom.

6. Carefully flip the scallops (try not to break them!), and sear for 1 to 2 minutes, or until they are starting to brown.

7. Add the lemon zest, the juice of 1 lemon, the thyme, ½ cup of parsley, a pinch each of salt and pepper, and the water. Mix everything, and bring the liquid to a simmer. Poach the scallops for 4 to 5 minutes, or until just cooked through and slightly opaque. Scallops cook quickly and become tough and chewy if overcooked, so remove from the heat as soon as they appear opaque. Leaving the poaching liquid in the pan, transfer the scallops to a plate, and cover them to keep warm.

8. To make the sauce, increase the heat to medium-high, and let the poaching liquid reduce to about two-thirds of the original volume. Remove from the heat.

9. To serve, in a large bowl, toss the potatoes with the remaining 2 tablespoons of oil and a pinch of salt. Press the potatoes using a fork, and transfer to serving plates.

10. Serve the scallops over the potatoes. Drizzle the sauce and remaining lemon juice on top, and add a pinch of parsley for color.

Beyond the basics: *For an even tastier, but a little less healthy version, substitute white wine for the 2 cups water.*

Per Serving: Calories: 467; Total fat: 15g; Carbohydrates: 51g; Fiber: 6g; Protein: 33g; Sodium: 857mg

Lemon-Tarragon Salmon and Roasted Broccolini

SERVES 4 / ACTIVE TIME: 20 MINUTES

DAIRY-FREE, GLUTEN-FREE

Salmon is always a good choice for a meal that is simple, delicious, and rich in omega-3s, protein, and vitamins. Lemon and tarragon bring out a warm and citrusy flavor profile. The salmon will melt in your mouth, and the broccolini adds a bit of crunch and texture.

1½ cups brown rice, preferably basmati

Pinch sea salt, plus ½ teaspoon

1½ cups coconut milk

1½ cups water

3 tablespoons fresh tarragon leaves, chopped

3 garlic cloves, minced

1 tablespoon Dijon mustard

¼ teaspoon freshly ground black pepper

2 tablespoons light olive oil

2 tablespoons freshly squeezed lemon juice (½ lemon)

2 pounds skinless salmon, cut into 4 fillets

2 pounds broccolini, rinsed and leaves trimmed

1 recipe SPOOG (page 18)

1 large lemon, quartered

1. Preheat the oven to 400°F. Line a baking sheet with parchment paper.

2. In a medium pot, combine the rice, a pinch of salt, the coconut milk, and water. Bring to a boil.

3. Reduce the heat to maintain a simmer. Cover the pot with a tight-fitting lid, and cook for 50 minutes, or until the liquid has been absorbed and the rice is soft. Refrain from removing the lid while cooking to check the rice. Remove from the heat. Let rest, covered, until serving.

4. Meanwhile, to make the marinade, in a medium bowl, stir together the tarragon, garlic, mustard, remaining ½ teaspoon of salt, the pepper, oil, and lemon juice.

5. Put the salmon in an oven-safe casserole dish, and pour in the marinade, turning the salmon to coat. Refrigerate for about 30 minutes to marinate (not too long, or the lemon juice will start to "cook" the salmon).

6. On the prepared baking sheet, toss the broccolini and SPOOG, then spread it out.

7. Transfer the baking sheet to the oven, and bake for 10 to 15 minutes, or until the broccolini is crisp on the outer pieces and tender in the middle. Remove from the oven.

8. At the same time, transfer the casserole dish to the oven, and bake the salmon for 10 to 12 minutes, or until just barely cooked through. The salmon will turn from bright pink on the outside to a light, opaque white color. The internal temperature should be between 110°F and 140°F. Remove from the oven.

9. Plate the salmon on top of the rice, and drizzle any remaining marinade on top. Serve with the broccolini and lemon quarters on the side. Squeeze the lemon juice on top just before eating.

Healthy swap: *If you can't find tarragon, fresh sage or fresh basil is a great substitute. Broccoli can also replace the broccolini if it is unavailable.*

Per Serving: Calories: 920; Total fat: 46g; Carbohydrates: 75g; Fiber: 9g; Protein: 59g; Sodium: 448mg

Linguine with Lemon-Sage Chicken, English Peas, and Pecorino

SERVES 4 / ACTIVE TIME: 30 MINUTES

NUT-FREE

Peas and pecorino are a classic Italian combination. This recipe combines them with pasta and chicken for a creamy, comforting meal. Sage is an herb I grow in my garden. It grows very easily and loves to take over the garden if I let it.

Sea salt

1 pound linguine

3 tablespoons olive oil, divided

½ yellow onion, chopped

4 garlic cloves, minced

2 pounds boneless, skinless chicken breasts or thighs, cut into 2-inch pieces

Freshly ground black pepper

1 (8½-ounce) can English peas, drained, or frozen peas, thawed

2 tablespoons balsamic vinegar

Juice of ½ lemon

1 tablespoon fresh sage leaves, minced

4 ounces Pecorino Romano or parmesan cheese, shaved

1. Bring a large pot of salted water to a boil. Cook the linguine according to the package instructions until very al dente (still with a slight bite, not completely soft). Drain the linguine, and return it to the pot.

2. Add 2 tablespoons of oil, and toss.

3. Preheat a large skillet over medium-high heat.

4. When the skillet is hot, drizzle in the remaining 1 tablespoon of oil, and add the onion. Sauté for about 2 minutes, or until the onion is translucent.

5. Add the garlic, and cook for 30 seconds, or until fragrant.

6. Season the chicken with salt and pepper. Add the chicken to the skillet. Cook for 5 to 7 minutes, stirring every couple of minutes, or until browned and cooked through.

7. Add the peas, vinegar, lemon juice, and sage. Cook for 1 minute, or until the peas and vinegar have caramelized.

8. Add the linguine, and toss to combine. Cook for 1 to 2 minutes, or until the linguine is hot. Remove from the heat.

9. Serve the pasta immediately, topped with the cheese.

Healthy swap: *Give gluten-free pasta a try, such as one made from chickpeas, lentils, quinoa, or brown rice.*

Per Serving: Calories: 924; Total fat: 24g; Carbohydrates: 98g; Fiber: 6g; Protein: 75g; Sodium: 677mg

Lamb Steak and Roasted Vegetables

SERVES 4 / ACTIVE TIME: 20 MINUTES

DAIRY-FREE, GLUTEN-FREE, NUT-FREE

If I am cooking for a crowd, this is a simple go-to that impresses without being difficult to prepare. Lamb is a delicious way to get in your protein and iron, as well as some anti-inflammatory compounds. Lamb is also full of omega-3s, which are great for brain and eye health. Lamb reminds me of hiking the hills of New Zealand and then dining on the freshest of lamb. I hope this recipe transports you to somewhere exciting, too!

2 pounds lamb loin or lamb leg steaks

1 teaspoon garlic powder

Sea salt

Freshly ground black pepper

1 bunch asparagus

1 pound cauliflower, broccoli or romanesco (about 1 head), cut into small florets

2 fennel bulbs, cored and cut into thin strips

4 to 6 large carrots, peeled and cut on a bias into thirds

3 tablespoons olive oil, divided

4 garlic cloves

2 tablespoons chopped fresh tarragon leaves

1 (14-ounce) can green peas, drained

1. Preheat the oven to 400°F. Line a baking sheet with parchment paper.

2. Rub the lamb all over with the garlic powder, salt, and pepper.

3. Snap each asparagus spear at the natural breaking point, which is usually about halfway up. Discard the bottoms, which are not very edible. Cut the spears in half so that they are about the length of your finger.

4. In a large bowl, toss together the asparagus, cauliflower, fennel, carrots, 2 tablespoons of oil, the garlic, tarragon, and a pinch each of salt and pepper.

5. Spread the vegetables out on the prepared baking sheet.

6. Transfer the baking sheet to the oven, and roast for about 15 minutes.

7. Stir the vegetables, using a spatula, then spread the peas out all over the vegetables. Roast for 5 to 10 minutes, or until the vegetables are browned on the outside and soft on the inside. Remove from the oven.

8. While the vegetables are cooking, preheat a skillet over medium-high heat.

9. When the skillet is hot, drizzle in the remaining 1 tablespoon of oil.

10. Add the lamb, and sear the outside for about 5 minutes on one side, or until browned.

11. Flip the lamb, and sear the other side for 5 minutes, or until browned.

12. Flip the lamb again. Reduce the heat to medium-low. Cover the pan, and cook for 5 to 10 minutes, or until the lamb is firmer to the touch. When a thermometer is inserted into the lamb, it should read 135°F to 140°F (the lamb will continue to cook when resting). Turn off the heat. Cover with aluminum foil, and let sit for 10 minutes.

13. Transfer the lamb to a cutting board. Thinly slice.

14. Pour the vegetables into a big bowl to serve, and fold in the lamb strips. Serve hot.

Beyond the basics: *Try adding 2 pounds Yukon Gold potatoes to this mix to make it a little heartier. Rinse the potatoes, cut them in half, and toss them in 2 recipes SPOOG. Try adding 1 tablespoon chopped rosemary for some more flavor. Roast on a baking sheet for 30 to 40 minutes while prepping the remaining ingredients in this recipe. Fold into the final bowl of vegetables and lamb.*

Per Serving: Calories: 725; Total fat: 44g; Carbohydrates: 33g; Fiber: 9g; Protein: 51g; Sodium: 487mg

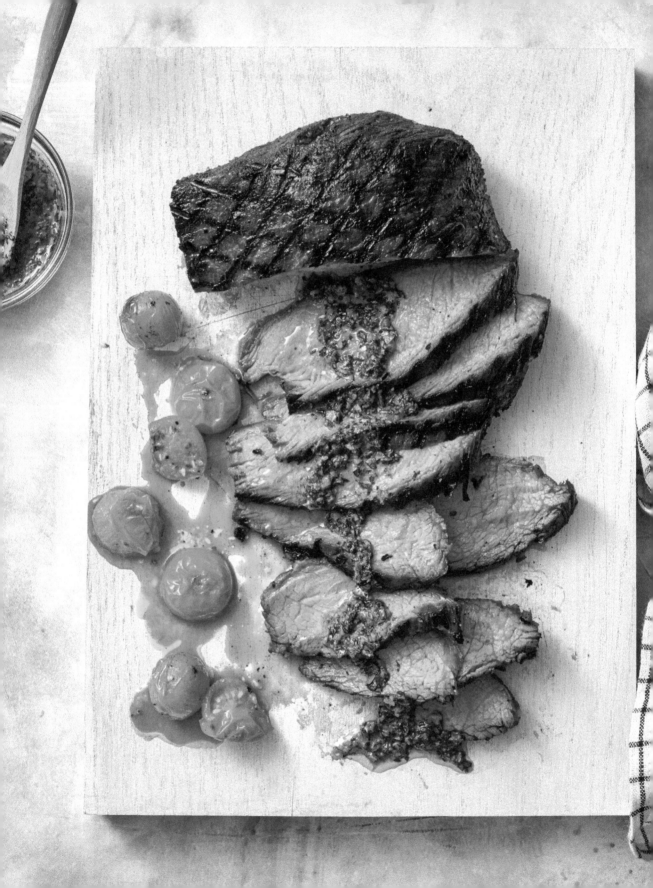

Grilled Tri-Tip with Chimichurri

SERVES 4 / ACTIVE TIME: 20 MINUTES

DAIRY-FREE, GLUTEN-FREE, NUT-FREE

Chimichurri goes with almost anything—meats, fish, grains, eggs, and more! It is similar to pesto and can be made using different types of herbs and spices, but in this recipe we'll use a combination of cilantro, parsley, garlic, and more to create the perfect pairing for grilled tri-tip. This recipe is one I learned from one of my favorite chefs, Melanie.

½ cup liquid aminos or low-sodium soy sauce

⅓ cup freshly squeezed orange juice (about 1 orange)

2 tablespoons maple syrup

8 recipes SPOOG (page 18), divided, plus more olive oil as needed

2 pounds beef tri-tip

¼ cup red-wine vinegar

¼ cup minced fresh cilantro

¼ cup minced fresh flat-leaf parsley

2 large garlic cloves, peeled

½ shallot, chopped

½ Fresno or serrano chile, seeded and finely chopped

½ teaspoon sea salt, plus more as needed

1. In a large container with a lid, combine the liquid aminos, orange juice, maple syrup, and 4 recipes of SPOOG.

2. Add the tri-tip, cover, and let sit at room temperature for at least 1 hour, or refrigerate for 4 to 12 hours before cooking.

3. To make the chimichurri, in a blender or food processor, combine the vinegar, remaining 4 recipes of SPOOG, the cilantro, parsley, garlic, shallot, chile, and salt, adding more oil if needed to loosen the mixture. Blend into a finely processed green sauce.

4. Preheat a grill to 500°F. Line a plate with aluminum foil.

5. Put the tri-tip on the grill, and sear on each side for 5 to 6 minutes, or until dark grill marks appear.

>>

6. Reduce the heat to medium. Cover the grill, and cook for about 5 minutes, depending on the thickness of the meat, or until it reaches an internal temperature of 125°F for rare, 130°F for medium-rare, or 135°F for medium. You want the meat to still be slightly rare on the inside, depending on your preference, knowing the meat will continue to cook while it rests. Remove from the heat. Transfer to the prepared plate, cover with foil, and let rest for 10 minutes.

7. Slice the tri-tip, and serve with the chimichurri on top.

Beyond the basics: *Give this dish some extra color by slicing some cherry tomatoes or sun-dried tomatoes, heating them in a skillet over medium-high heat with a bit of olive oil for about 2 minutes, and pouring them on top of the tri-tip with the chimichurri.*

Per Serving: Calories: 536; Total fat: 32g; Carbohydrates: 14g; Fiber: 1g; Protein: 50g; Sodium: 1,099mg

Moroccan-Style Chicken Thighs with Dried Plums over Brown Rice

SERVES 4 / ACTIVE TIME: 20 MINUTES

DAIRY-FREE, GLUTEN-FREE, NUT-FREE

Dried plums add a subtle sweetness to this dish, complementing the healing spices of cinnamon, ginger, paprika, and garlic powder that coat the chicken. Simmering the chicken over low heat will make the meat very tender and bring out all the bright flavors—it might just transport you to Morocco!

1 cup brown rice

4 cups low-sodium chicken broth, divided

Sea salt

2 pounds chicken thighs (with or without skin and bones)

1 tablespoon extra-virgin olive oil

Freshly ground black pepper

2 tablespoons ground cinnamon, divided

3 teaspoons garlic powder, divided

3 teaspoons ground ginger, divided

1 teaspoon smoked paprika, divided

1 cup white wine

1 cup dried plums, prunes, or apricots

1. In a medium pot, combine the rice, 2 cups of broth, and a pinch of salt. Bring to a boil.

2. Reduce the heat to maintain a low simmer. Cover the pot with a tight-fitting lid, and cook for 50 minutes, or until the broth has been absorbed and the rice is soft. Refrain from removing the lid while cooking to check the rice. Remove from the heat. Let rest, covered, until serving.

3. Preheat a large skillet with a lid over medium-high heat.

4. Pat the chicken dry.

5. Pour the oil into the skillet, and tilt to coat the bottom.

6. Immediately add the chicken, and sear on one side for 3 to 5 minutes, or until browned but not cooked through.

7. While searing, generously sprinkle salt and pepper on the uncooked side of the chicken and 1 tablespoon of cinnamon, 1½ teaspoons of garlic powder, 1½ teaspoons of ginger, and ½ teaspoon of paprika.

8. Using tongs, flip the chicken, and sear the other side for 2 to 3 minutes. Sprinkle with salt, pepper, and the remaining 1 tablespoon of cinnamon, 1½ teaspoons of garlic powder, 1½ teaspoons of ginger, and ½ teaspoon of paprika.

9. Pour in the wine and remaining 2 cups of broth.

10. Spread the plums over the chicken and in the broth. Bring the liquid to a boil.

11. Reduce the heat to medium-low. Cover the skillet, and simmer for 20 to 30 minutes, or until the chicken has cooked through with no pink remaining and the internal temperature reaches 165°F. Remove from the heat.

12. Serve the chicken hot on top of a scoop of brown rice with the dried plums and juices on top.

Healthy swap: *For a leaner version, use chicken breast or a combination of breasts and thighs. For a vegetarian version, substitute large portobello mushrooms for the chicken and low-sodium vegetable broth for the chicken broth.*

Per Serving: Calories: 626; Total fat: 14g; Carbohydrates: 64g; Fiber: 7g; Protein: 50g; Sodium: 265mg

Grilled Plant-Based Burgers with Avocado-Goat Cheese Spread

SERVES 4 / ACTIVE TIME: 20 MINUTES

VEGETARIAN

Using a plant-based protein, such as ground "beef," is an amazing way to eat a hearty, satisfying, delicious, nutritious meal. These new-age burgers have 19 grams of protein (or more) per serving, the same amount as beef from cattle. And they significantly reduce the environmental impact of the food's production versus raising and processing cattle. Even if you're not vegetarian, you can try incorporating them into your diet for a healthy balance.

1½ pounds ground plant-based burger meat

½ red onion, diced

¼ cup finely chopped fresh herbs, such as dill, cilantro, and parsley

2 recipes SPOOG (page 18), plus more sea salt as needed

½ teaspoon ground cumin

¼ teaspoon cayenne pepper

1 large ripe avocado

8 ounces goat cheese

2 tablespoons Dijon mustard

8 nutty seedy bread slices or 4 large romaine lettuce leaves (for a lettuce wrap instead)

1 large roma tomato, thinly cut into rounds

1. Preheat a grill to at least 550°F.

2. In a large bowl, using your hands, mix together the burger meat, onion, herbs, SPOOG, cumin, and cayenne until well incorporated.

3. Divide the meat into 4 to 6 balls, and press them down into thick, disk-like patties.

4. Halve the avocado, remove the pit (see page 151), and using a spoon, scoop the avocado meat into a small bowl.

5. Add the cheese and a pinch of salt. Using a fork, mash together the avocado and cheese.

6. Put the patties on the grill. Close the lid, and cook for 4 to 5 minutes, or until browned on the first side (being careful not to burn them).

7. Flip the patties, and cook for 4 to 5 minutes, or until cooked through and no longer pink.

>>

8. During the last 2 minutes of grilling, spread the mustard onto one side of each bread slice. Place the bread, mustard-side up, on the grill. Toast for 2 minutes, or until they have a slight crunch but are still tender in the middle. Remove from the heat.

9. Stack the burgers in this order: bread slice (or lettuce leaf), patty, scoop of avocado–goat cheese, tomato slice, and another slice of bread.

Beyond the basics: *Give your burger a boost by adding sautéed bell peppers or onions (see page 37) on top. Or finely chop ½ fresh ripe peach, and incorporate it into the burger mixture. It is delicious and adds moisture to your patty.*

Per Serving: Calories: 773; Total fat: 40g; Carbohydrates: 63g; Fiber: 16g; Protein: 46g; Sodium: 1,344mg

Mediterranean White Wine–Poached Halibut with Gnocchi

SERVES 4 / ACTIVE TIME: 35 MINUTES

DAIRY-FREE, NUT-FREE

When I think of some of the best, most delicious meals I've had, I always land on Mediterranean cuisine. I'm inspired by the bounty of fresh herbs, variety of vegetables, and light proteins, such as fish.

½ teaspoon sea salt, plus more for the cooking water

2 pounds halibut, cut into 4 fillets

½ teaspoon freshly ground black pepper

4 tablespoons extra-virgin olive oil, divided

½ red onion, diced

8 garlic cloves, minced

½ cup dry white wine

2 cups low-sodium vegetable broth or chicken broth

Grated zest of 3 large lemons

Juice of 3 large lemons, plus more for serving

10 large fresh basil leaves, stacked and thinly sliced

1 pound frozen gnocchi

1. Fill a medium pot with water, and add a couple pinches of salt. Bring to a boil.

2. Season the halibut fillets all over with the salt and pepper. Set aside at room temperature for 10 minutes, or refrigerate until you are ready to cook.

3. Preheat a large skillet over medium-high heat.

4. When the skillet is hot, drizzle in 2 tablespoons of oil.

5. Reduce the heat to medium. Add the onion, and sauté for 2 to 3 minutes, or until translucent.

6. Add the garlic, and cook for 30 seconds, or until fragrant and starting to turn translucent. Do not let it turn brown and burn.

7. Add the wine, broth, lemon zest, lemon juice, and basil. Bring to a boil.

8. Reduce the heat to medium-low to bring the liquid to a simmer. Add the halibut, and cover the skillet.

9. Reduce the heat to low. Poach for 8 to 10 minutes, or until the halibut is semi-firm to the touch, white, and flaky. Remove from the heat.

>>

10. As soon as you add the halibut to the poaching liquid, pour the gnocchi into the boiling water, and cook according to the package instructions. Drain.

11. Drizzle the gnocchi with the remaining 2 tablespoons of oil, and stir so they don't stick together. Cover until the halibut is ready.

12. Scoop a helping of gnocchi into a bowl. Place a halibut fillet on top, and drizzle with some of the poaching liquid.

13. Squeeze fresh lemon juice on top, and serve hot.

Healthy swap: *For a healthier grain option, serve with forbidden black rice, cooked farro, or cooked quinoa instead of gnocchi.*

Per Serving: Calories: 434; Total fat: 14g; Carbohydrates: 26g; Fiber: 2g; Protein: 45g; Sodium: 718mg

Farro Risotto with Garlic, Thyme, and White Beans

SERVES 4 / ACTIVE TIME: 35 MINUTES

NUT-FREE, VEGETARIAN

This rich, creamy risotto uses farro instead of the traditional Arborio rice for a slightly heartier consistency. Originally from northern Italy, risotto is a rice dish cooked in broth until it is thick and creamy. It is important to add the liquid incrementally and to stir frequently so the grain has time to release its starches, creating a thick consistency. This comforting dish is often associated with fancy restaurants, but really, it's just home cooking.

2 cups low-sodium vegetable broth

1 tablespoon extra-virgin olive oil

½ red onion, diced

3 garlic cloves, minced

1 teaspoon dried thyme

1 cup pearled farro, rinsed

1 cup dry white wine

1 bay leaf

1 cup canned no-salt-added cannellini beans, drained and rinsed

4 ounces Pecorino Romano or parmesan cheese, finely grated

8 fresh basil leaves, stacked and thinly sliced

1. In a small pot, bring the broth to a gentle boil over medium heat, then cover the pot and turn off the heat.

2. Preheat a medium pot over medium-high heat.

3. When the pot is hot, drizzle in the oil, and add the onion.

4. Reduce the heat to medium. Cook for about 2 minutes, or until the onion starts to turn translucent.

5. Add the garlic and thyme. Cook for 1 minute, or until fragrant and the garlic is starting to turn slightly translucent.

6. Stir in the farro. Cook for 1 minute, or until toasted.

7. Stir in the wine, and add the bay leaf. Cook, stirring often, for 3 to 4 minutes, or until the wine has been absorbed.

>>

8. Pour in ½ cup of the warm broth. Cook, stirring, until absorbed into the farro. Add ½ cup more broth, and cook, stirring often, until absorbed. The farro should take about 20 minutes to cook and may require more broth to become soft and tender.

9. Once the farro is cooked, stir in the beans and cheese. Remove from the heat and discard the bay leaf.

10. Serve the risotto garnished with the basil.

Make it healthier: *When buying canned beans, look for "no-salt-added" beans to control the salt level in your food. Excess sodium can cause bloating, weight gain, and high blood pressure.*

Per Serving: Calories: 445; Total fat: 12g; Carbohydrates: 58g; Fiber: 11g; Protein: 18g; Sodium: 523mg

Turmeric Vegetable "Paella"

SERVES 4 / ACTIVE TIME: 20 MINUTES

- -
DAIRY-FREE, GLUTEN-FREE, NUT-FREE, VEGETARIAN
- -

The roots of this recipe stem from one of my favorite cookbook authors. I've made adjustments over time to make it my own (and better—in my opinion!). It delivers a hearty vegan meal that is full of flavor, fiber, and color. Some people claim that "paella" is not "paella" without meat, but this is made using the traditional paella method.

2 cups vegetable stock

2 recipes SPOOG (page 18), divided, plus more olive oil for drizzling

½ yellow onion, diced

2 bay leaves

½ teaspoon ground turmeric

¼ teaspoon smoked paprika

1 cup Arborio rice

½ cup white wine

½ cup cherry tomatoes, halved

¼ cup chopped canned artichokes

Juice of 1 lemon

½ cup chopped fresh parsley

1. In a small pot, bring the stock to a light boil over high heat, then cover the pot and turn off the heat.

2. Preheat a wide pot or high-sided skillet over medium-high heat.

3. When the pot is hot, drizzle in 1 tablespoon of oil, and add the onion. Sauté for 3 to 4 minutes, or until translucent.

4. Stir in 1 recipe of SPOOG, the bay leaves, turmeric, and paprika to coat the onion. Cook for 1 minute to activate the flavor of the spices.

5. Add the rice, and stir-fry to coat the grains in the spices.

6. Pour in the wine, and cook for about 1 minute, or until the rice has absorbed the wine.

7. Pour the hot stock over the rice. Give the pot a good shake to even out the stock and loosen the rice from the bottom.

8. Reduce the heat to a low simmer. Gently cook, without stirring, for about 15 minutes, or until most of the liquid has been absorbed.

9. Scatter the tomatoes over the rice, and let them steam from the remaining stock for about 5 minutes.

>>

10. Scatter the artichokes over the rice.

11. Increase the heat to medium-high. Cook for 1 to 2 minutes, or until the rice on the bottom of the pot is toasted. Turn off the heat. Taste, and drizzle the remaining 1 recipe of SPOOG on top for extra flavor. Tightly cover the pot with a lid or aluminum foil, and steam for 10 more minutes to finish cooking.

12. When ready to serve, discard the bay leaves, sprinkle the lemon juice on top, and garnish with the parsley.

Make it easier: *Add the tomatoes, artichokes, lemon juice, and parsley to the rice with the hot stock. Stir, then cook for about 25 minutes without stirring, or until the liquid has been absorbed.*

Per Serving: Calories: 280; Total fat: 7g; Carbohydrates: 44g; Fiber: 3g; Protein: 4g; Sodium: 361mg

Turkey Meatballs with Warm Spinach Yogurt

SERVES 4 / ACTIVE TIME: 30 MINUTES

My mother used to make turkey meatballs when I was a kid. This is a version I learned while traveling in London. London has all sorts of exquisite Mediterranean restaurants. The yogurt in this dish brings out a soft, tender flavor in the turkey.

½ yellow onion, finely chopped

3 recipes SPOOG (page 18), divided, plus more olive oil for sautéing

2 pounds ground turkey (half lean, half dark meat)

½ cup oat flour or all-purpose flour, plus more as needed

2½ teaspoons ground cumin

¼ cup fresh cilantro, finely chopped

1 large egg

3 cups coarsely chopped fresh spinach

Juice of ½ lemon

2 cups plain, full-fat Greek yogurt

Pinch cayenne pepper

1. Preheat the oven to 425°F. Line a baking sheet with parchment paper.

2. Preheat a heavy sauté pan or skillet over high heat.

3. Put the onion and 1 recipe of SPOOG in the pan. Sauté for 2 to 3 minutes, or until darkly browned. Remove from the heat. Let cool.

4. In a large bowl, combine the turkey, onion, 1 recipe of SPOOG, the flour, cumin, cilantro, and egg. If the mixture seems very goopy, add more flour until it holds together enough to form a ball. Mix well using your hands.

5. Shape the mixture into 12 to 16 balls, about the size of golf balls.

6. Put the meatballs on the prepared baking sheet.

7. Transfer the baking sheet to the oven, and cook for about 10 minutes.

8. Reduce the oven temperature to 375°F.

9. Let the meatballs cook for another 5 minutes, or until the meat bounces back when you press a meatball using your finger. If you are unsure if they are done, break one open to check that it is no longer pink, or use a thermometer. A thermometer inserted into the middle of the meatball should read 160°F to 165°F. Remove from the oven.

>>

10. While the meatballs are cooking, preheat a small pot over medium heat.

11. Drizzle in about 1 tablespoon of oil, and add the spinach. Stir the spinach slowly, allowing it to wilt.

12. Add the lemon juice, yogurt, cayenne, and remaining 1 recipe of SPOOG.

13. Reduce the heat to low. Stir until the sauce is warm and fully combined. If needed, stir in 1 to 2 tablespoons of water to make the sauce a little thinner. Remove from the heat.

14. Serve the sauce immediately over the hot meatballs.

Make it easier: *Skip making the full yogurt sauce, and instead top the meatballs with fresh yogurt.*

Per Serving: Calories: 610; Total fat: 36g; Carbohydrates: 25g; Fiber: 2g; Protein: 51g; Sodium: 774mg

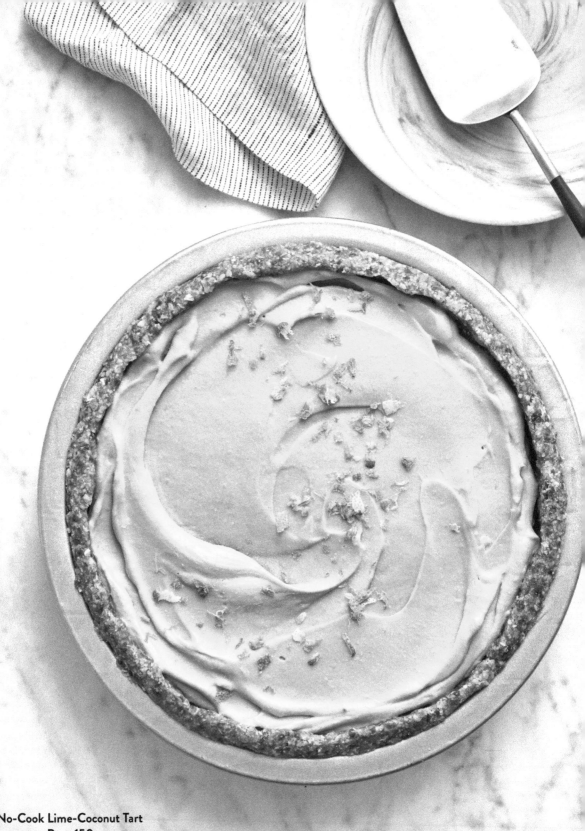

No-Cook Lime-Coconut Tart
Page 150

CHAPTER ELEVEN

DESSERTS

- - - - -

Summer Peach Clafoutis with Lemon-Honey Crème Fraîche

SERVES 4 / ACTIVE TIME: 15 MINUTES

VEGETARIAN

Clafoutis is a simple and incredibly delicious custard-like dessert from France. Traditionally, it is made with cherries, but you can use any type of fruit you please. This version highlights summer stone fruit paired with a delightfully sweet and slightly sour crème fraîche.

Coconut oil, for coating the casserole dish

1¼ cups almond milk

⅔ cup coconut sugar

3 large eggs

1 tablespoon vanilla extract

⅛ teaspoon sea salt

1 cup all-purpose flour or gluten-free 1:1 flour

2 generous cups coarsely chopped fresh ripe peaches

½ cup honey

Grated zest of 1 lemon

1 cup crème fraîche or plain, full-fat Greek yogurt

1. Preheat the oven to 375°F. Using a paper towel, generously coat the bottom and sides of a 9-by-9-inch casserole dish (at least 1½ inches deep) with coconut oil.

2. In a medium bowl, whisk together the almond milk, sugar, eggs, vanilla, and salt until smooth.

3. Slowly whisk in the flour a little at a time until you have a thin, flan-like batter. Pour into the prepared casserole dish.

4. Sprinkle the peaches all over the batter.

5. Transfer the casserole dish to the oven, and bake for 30 to 35 minutes, or until lightly browned on the outside and the edges have set. Remove from the oven. Let rest for at least 15 minutes.

6. Meanwhile, in a medium bowl, whisk together the honey and lemon zest to blend.

7. Fold in the crème fraîche.

8. Serve the clafoutis with a dollop of lemon-honey crème fraîche on top.

Make it easier: *Skip the crème fraîche, and sprinkle coconut sugar on top of the clafoutis after cooling, or serve with whipped cream or ice cream.*

Per Serving: Calories: 475; Total fat: 8g; Carbohydrates: 91g; Fiber: 2g; Protein: 11g; Sodium: 211mg

Anja's Dark Chocolate–Berry Crumble

SERVES 3 OR 4 / ACTIVE TIME: 15 MINUTES

GLUTEN-FREE, VEGETARIAN

This is my FAVORITE recipe of all time. After a lot of testing, I've figured out my favorite ratios. I make this every time I have guests, and they always beg to eat it again and again. And who knew it was a clean, healthy dessert, too!

1 cup fresh strawberries, cut into bite-size pieces

1 cup fresh blueberries

2 tablespoons coconut sugar

1 teaspoon sea salt, divided

¾ cup almond flour

¼ cup coconut oil

¼ cup honey

½ teaspoon vanilla extract

6 ounces dark chocolate (preferably at least 80 percent cocoa), chopped into small pieces

¼ cup shaved coconut

1. Preheat the oven to 375°F.

2. In a medium bowl, toss together the strawberries, blueberries, sugar, and ½ teaspoon of salt to combine.

3. In a large bowl, using clean hands, combine the flour, oil, honey, vanilla, and remaining ½ teaspoon of salt, mixing well until no longer clumpy and everything combines well to make a crumble.

4. Pour the berries into an 8-by-8-inch casserole dish, and spread them across the bottom.

5. Sprinkle the chocolate on top, followed by the crumble mixture.

6. Transfer the casserole dish to the oven, and bake for 15 to 20 minutes, or until the crumble starts to brown. Remove from the oven, leaving the oven on.

7. Sprinkle the coconut on top. Return the casserole dish to the oven, and bake for 3 minutes, or until the coconut is slightly toasted. Remove from the oven. Serve hot.

Beyond the basics: *Refrigerate a 13½-ounce can of coconut cream for at least 2 hours. Open the can, and scoop the top layer of cream into a bowl. Save the coconut water for another use. Add 1 tablespoon coconut sugar, ½ teaspoon vanilla extract, and ½ teaspoon sea salt to the cream. Using an electric mixer, whip the cream until peaks form. Serve the coconut whipped cream on top of the crumble.*

Per Serving: Calories: 796; Total fat: 55g; Carbohydrates: 72g; Fiber: 12g; Protein: 10g; Sodium: 559mg

No-Cook Lime-Coconut Tart

SERVES 6 TO 8 / ACTIVE TIME: 20 MINUTES

DAIRY-FREE, GLUTEN-FREE, VEGETARIAN

This zesty tart is my spin on key lime pie. It's dairy-free and doesn't require any baking. Key lime pie is a quintessentially American dessert that makes me think of my good friend Liz. She is well known for making "healthier" desserts, and she made me weak with a key lime pie recently. She didn't give me the recipe, but here is what I would expect it to look like.

1 cup raw almonds or pecans, soaked in water for 8 hours, drained

¼ cup unsweetened shredded coconut

1 cup medjool dates, pitted

1 teaspoon sea salt, divided

3 ripe avocados

¼ cup maple syrup, plus more as needed

1½ tablespoons coconut oil, melted and cooled

¼ cup freshly squeezed lime juice (about 2 limes), plus more as needed

Grated zest of 1 lime

1. Line a 9-inch pie tin with parchment paper.

2. In a food processor, pulse the almonds until they are in tiny pieces.

3. Add the coconut, dates, and ½ teaspoon of salt. Pulse until a dough-like ball forms that can be squeezed into one big dough ball.

4. Press the dough into the prepared pie tin like a crust, over the bottom and up the sides. Freeze for 1 hour to harden.

5. Meanwhile, make the filling: halve the avocados, remove the pits (see Beyond the basics tip), and using a spoon, scoop the avocado meat into the food processor.

6. Add the maple syrup, oil, lime juice, and remaining ½ teaspoon of salt. Process on high speed until smooth. Taste, and add more maple syrup if you want it sweeter. If the avocados are too ripe, add more lime juice to hide the overripe flavor.

7. Remove the piecrust from the freezer. Spread the filling into the crust, and using a spoon, smooth the top.

8. Sprinkle the lime zest on top.

9. Put the pie back into the freezer for at least 2 hours to harden. Remove the pie from the freezer 15 to 20 minutes before serving to soften.

Beyond the basics: *When pitting an avocado, halve the avocado lengthwise, and twist to separate. Place the halves on a cutting board, pit-side up. Wedge a sharp knife into the pit (be careful that your fingers are nowhere nearby—the pit is slippery, and your knife can slip!), then use the knife to twist the pit out of the flesh. Toss the pit. Now your avocado is ready to slice and scoop out of the skin using a spoon.*

Per Serving: Calories: 487; Total fat: 31g; Carbohydrates: 53g; Fiber: 12g; Protein: 9g; Sodium: 280mg

Cinnamon-Poached Pears with Chocolate Sauce

SERVES 4 / ACTIVE TIME: 20 MINUTES

GLUTEN-FREE, NUT-FREE, VEGETARIAN

This autumn dessert will warm your taste buds and fill your kitchen with scents of cinnamon and melted dark chocolate. There are many variations on poached pears, such as the classic Poires à la Beaujolaise, *or pears poached in red wine, and pears poached with different combinations of cardamom, ginger, lemon zest, and vanilla, perhaps with a side of crème anglaise. Take your pick; you can't go wrong.*

4 cups water

1 cup freshly squeezed orange juice

½ cup honey

4 cinnamon sticks

2 teaspoons vanilla extract

½ teaspoon sea salt

4 firm pears, Bosc or another type

8 ounces dark chocolate (70 percent cocoa or higher), chopped

1. In a medium pot, combine the water, orange juice, honey, cinnamon sticks, vanilla, and salt. Bring to a boil over high heat.

2. Halve the pears lengthwise, and using a spoon, remove the core. Put the pear halves into the boiling liquid.

3. Reduce the heat to a simmer. Cover the pot, and simmer, spooning the cooking liquid over the pears every few minutes and rotating them often, for about 20 minutes, or until the pears are tender. If needed, let them simmer longer to become even softer.

4. Using a slotted spoon, remove the pears, and place them in a bowl.

5. Add the chocolate to the simmering liquid to melt, stirring continuously. Remove from the heat.

6. Serve the poached pears with the chocolate sauce on top.

Beyond the basics: *For a more French-style version, swap out the water for white wine, and follow the instructions as listed.*

Per Serving: Calories: 606; Total fat: 25g; Carbohydrates: 96g; Fiber: 12g; Protein: 6g; Sodium: 249mg

"Healthier" Deluxe Chocolate Chip Cookies

MAKES 16 TO 20 COOKIES / ACTIVE TIME: 20 MINUTES

GLUTEN-FREE, VEGETARIAN

My mom is a cookie fiend! She has been eating one chocolate chip cookie per day since I was in her belly. I do not have a metabolism like hers, but I definitely love them, too. So, I've created a gluten-free and refined sugar–free cookie that is crunchy on the outside, soft inside, and absolutely delicious. We fight over them in my house!

3 cups almond flour

¾ cup gluten-free 1:1 flour

¾ cup shredded unsweetened coconut

1½ teaspoons baking powder

¾ teaspoon fine sea salt

¾ cup honey

9 tablespoons coconut oil, melted

¼ cup coconut sugar

4 large eggs

1½ teaspoons vanilla extract

1 (12-ounce) bar 70 to 85 percent cocoa dark chocolate, chopped

1 cup chopped almonds, pecans, or hazelnuts

1. Preheat the oven to 375°F.

2. In a large bowl, using a wooden spoon, stir together the almond flour, gluten-free flour, shredded coconut, baking powder, and salt until well mixed.

3. In a medium bowl, whisk together the honey, coconut oil, coconut sugar, eggs, and vanilla until smooth.

4. To make the dough, using a wooden mixing spoon, little by little mix the dry ingredients into the wet ingredients.

5. Mix in the chocolate and almonds.

6. Wet your hands with cold water (which helps make smoother balls), and roll the dough into 16 to 20 balls, each a little bigger than a golf ball.

7. Place each ball on a baking sheet 1 inch apart.

>>

8. Transfer the baking sheet to the oven, and bake for 10 to 12 minutes, or just until the cookies start to settle and begin to brown on top. DO NOT overbake. You're better off under-baking these cookies. Extra gooey insides make them extra delicious. Remove from the oven.

Beyond the basics: *Make the dough ahead, roll it into a long log, and put it in a large tightly sealed container. Refrigerate until you're ready to bake, or for up to 3 days. When ready, cut the log into 1-inch-thick slices, and bake as directed.*

Per Serving (1 cookie): Calories: 338; Total fat: 24g; Carbohydrates: 28g; Fiber: 4g; Protein: 7g; Sodium: 89mg

Apricot, Honey, and Coconut Ice Cream

SERVES 4 / ACTIVE TIME: 10 MINUTES

DAIRY-FREE, GLUTEN-FREE, VEGETARIAN

Apricots are one of my favorite stone fruits! They're sweet, succulent, and a great source of fiber and vitamins. This summery dairy-free ice cream is exceptionally creamy thanks to the coconut cream and is just slightly sweetened with honey.

2 cups cashew milk

1 cup chopped summer apricots or peaches

1 cup coconut cream

⅓ cup honey, plus more as needed

½ teaspoon sea salt

Grated zest of ½ lemon

1. In a blender, combine the cashew milk, apricots, coconut cream, honey, salt, and lemon zest. Blend until smooth. Taste, and add more syrup if you like your ice cream sweeter.

2. Pour the mixture into a 9-by-5-inch metal bread pan, and smooth the top. Freeze for 2 hours.

3. Remove the pan from the freezer, and stir using a wooden spoon. Freeze again for 2 to 4 more hours. Remove from the freezer at least 15 minutes before serving to soften.

Beyond the basics: *If you don't have cashew milk, and you don't mind dairy, use Greek yogurt instead.*

Per Serving: Calories: 326; Total fat: 22g; Carbohydrates: 33g; Fiber: 2g; Protein: 3g; Sodium: 314mg

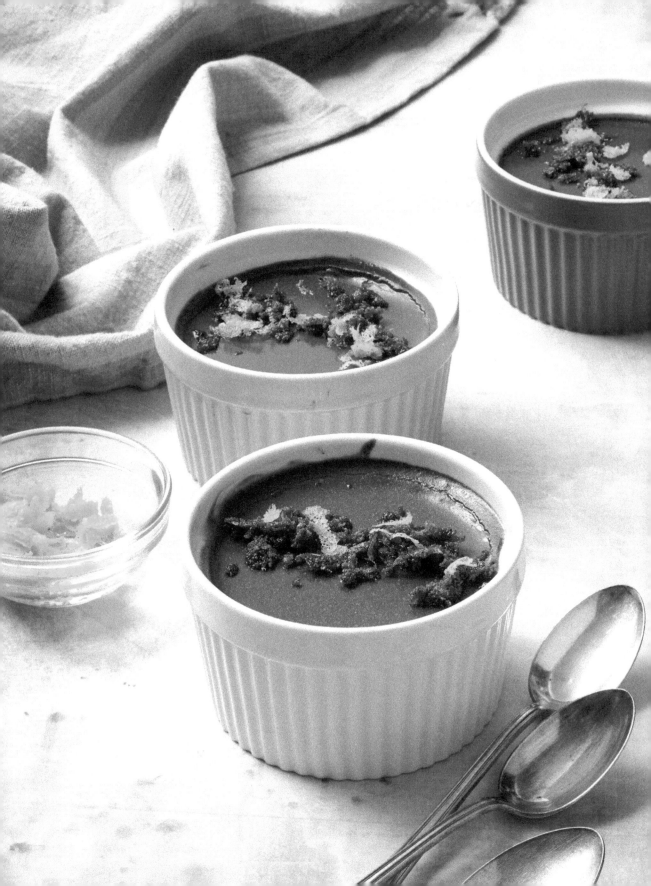

Orange-Chocolate Mousse with Citrus-Chili Sugar

SERVES 4 / ACTIVE TIME: 15 MINUTES

GLUTEN-FREE, VEGETARIAN

Orange adds a hint of sweet and tart to this rich chocolate mousse. And with a bit of orange zest and chili powder, you've got a perfect balance to the sweet, creamy chocolate centerpiece, with a little spice to kick it up a notch and rev up your metabolism.

2 cups full-fat coconut milk

¼ cup coconut oil

¼ cup maple syrup

1 teaspoon sea salt, divided

3 tablespoons freshly squeezed orange juice

8 ounces 70 to 85 percent cocoa dark chocolate, chopped

2 tablespoons coconut sugar

½ teaspoon chili powder

Grated zest of 1 orange

1. In a small pot, combine the coconut milk, oil, maple syrup, and ½ teaspoon of salt. Bring to a light boil over medium-high heat.

2. Reduce the heat to low. Simmer for 30 seconds to 1 minute.

3. Turn off the heat. Stir in the orange juice and chocolate, stirring constantly until the chocolate has fully melted. Transfer to a serving bowl or individual bowls, and refrigerate for at least 2 hours or overnight.

4. When ready to serve, in a small bowl, whisk together the sugar, chili powder, remaining ½ teaspoon of salt, and the orange zest to combine.

5. Remove the mousse from the refrigerator, and sprinkle the citrus-chili sugar on top.

Beyond the basics: *Try adding other spices to the chili sugar, instead of or in addition to the chili powder, such as cinnamon, cardamom, cayenne, nutmeg, or cloves.*

Per Serving: Calories: 754; Total fat: 62g; Carbohydrates: 48g; Fiber: 6g; Protein: 7g; Sodium: 447mg

QUICK REFERENCE GUIDE TO PREPPING AND COOKING VEGETABLES

PREPPING OPTIONS	TOOLS	RAW/ COOKED	COOKING METHODS	SERVING IDEAS
ASPARAGUS				
Remove bottom one-third of the stalk, at least, to remove more fibrous ends; peel into ribbons lengthwise, cut, or chop	Chef's knife, vegetable peeler	Raw/cooked	Roast, steam, sauté, simmer, slow cooker	Salad; add to pasta, legumes, grains, and vegetable dishes; soup; risotto; anything with eggs, such as quiche
AVOCADO				
Halve lengthwise, twist to separate, remove pit using a knife, cut into wedges or chunks; slide a spoon between the flesh and skin to scoop out; puree or mash	Chef's knife, spoon, fork	Raw/cooked	Grill, fry	Add to salads, sandwiches, and pasta; guacamole; place wedges on toast and top with olive oil, salt, and pepper; anything with cooked eggs, such as omelets; add to smoothies; use in a sauce or dressing
BEETS				
Slice off ends and peel; chop; dice; puree; peel into ribbons; grate	Chef's knife, paring knife, vegetable peeler, food processor or blender, box grater	Raw/cooked	Sauté, roast, simmer, steam, bake, slow cooker	As a chilled soup with sour cream and dill; add to salads, pasta, grains, and vegetable dishes; add puree to breads, ravioli filling; bake as chips; raw slaws; sauté with butter and maple syrup
BROCCOLI				
Trim fibrous ends and snap off leaves, peel off outer tough skin, separate florets by slicing through the stems; thinly slice the stems into long pieces or disks, chop, or dice	Chef's knife, vegetable peeler, food processor or blender	Raw/cooked	Bake, blanch, braise, fry, grill, roast, sauté, simmer, steam, stir-fry, slow cooker	Add to egg dishes such as casseroles and quiche; roast with olive oil, smoked paprika, salt, and pepper, and finish with lemon juice; stir-fry with other vegetables in sesame oil, and finish with soy sauce; add to raw salads, bowls, grains, legumes, and vegetable casseroles; roast and toss with pasta, lemon zest, grated parmesan cheese, and toasted bread crumbs; soup; add roasted broccoli to pizza toppings

PREPPING OPTIONS	TOOLS	RAW/ COOKED	COOKING METHODS	SERVING IDEAS
BRUSSELS SPROUTS				
Trim bottoms, and remove any wilted or yellowed leaves; thinly slice, halve, or grate	Chef's knife, food processor fitted with a grater	Raw/cooked	Roast, bake, steam, braise, fry, sauté, grill, slow cooker	Thinly slice or shred for raw salads; roast with apples; make a hash with potatoes, onion, and apple cider vinegar; toss with garlic, spices, and olive oil, and throw on the grill
CABBAGE				
Slice into wedges, thinly slice, or grate	Chef's knife, box grater	Raw/cooked	Roast, braise, sauté, steam, grill, bake, stir-fry, slow cooker	Roast wedges rubbed with olive oil, garlic paste, salt, and pepper; braise red cabbage with olive oil, apple cider vinegar, brown sugar, and apple chunks; slaw; cabbage rolls stuffed with rice and vegetables; pickle for kimchi; topping for tacos
CARROT				
Trim top and peel; slice, dice, grate, or peel into ribbons	Chef's knife, paring knife, box grater, vegetable peeler	Raw/cooked	Roast, braise, sauté, steam, grill, bake, stir-fry, slow cooker, simmer, steam	Raw in a salad; soup; slaw; soufflé; bread; cake; add to vegetable, grain, and legume dishes; simmer with butter, honey, and orange juice until all the liquid is gone except a glaze
CAULIFLOWER				
Trim bottom and remove leaves; slice from top to bottom into steaks; cut off florets at the stems; chop or dice stems; grate into rice, puree, or mash	Chef's knife, paring knife, box grater, food processor or blender	Raw/cooked	Bake, blanch, braise, grill, roast, sauté, simmer, steam, stir-fry, slow cooker	Puree into a sauce; grate into rice for risotto; roast whole, smothered with a spicy sauce; substitute for chicken in many dishes; soup; swap in for potatoes in mashed potatoes; toss with pasta, lemon, capers, and bread crumbs
CELERY				
Trim bottoms; cut into long strips or dice	Chef's knife	Raw/cooked	Roast, braise, sauté, bake, stir-fry, simmer	Use for making stock; braise in broth with tomatoes, onions, and top with shavings of parmesan; add to salads for crunch
CHILES (SERRANO, JALAPEÑO PEPPER)				
Trim off the stem, halve lengthwise, and remove the seeds and pith; slice, dice, or mince	Paring knife	Raw/cooked	Sauté, roast, bake, stir-fry	Roast with corn bread batter; roast with cheese; add to vegetable and legume dishes; add to cheese sandwiches or quesadillas; traditional tomato salsas or with diced pineapple

PREPPING OPTIONS	TOOLS	RAW/ COOKED	COOKING METHODS	SERVING IDEAS
CORN				
Remove kernels by standing a cob in a large bowl lined with a towel. Anchor it with one hand and slide a knife down the cob to slice off the kernels.	Chef's knife	Raw/cooked	Sauté, roast, simmer, steam, grill	Chowder; stew; add to tacos with black beans, tomatoes, and avocado with a squeeze of lime juice; sauté with pickled onion, basil, and tomatoes, then stuff into peppers with a little cheese; risotto; toss with thinly sliced vegetables, mint, and tomatoes; make Mexican corn
CUCUMBER				
Peel, halve, and scrape out pulpy seeds; cut into thin or thick slices, peel into long ribbons, dice, grate	Vegetable peeler, chef's knife, paring knife, spoon, box grater	Raw/cooked	Sauté, bake, stir-fry	Use in salads, especially Greek and Middle Eastern salads; swap out bread for cucumber disks; chilled soup; make a sandwich with cream cheese and dill; add slices to jugs of water; sauté with a little butter, salt, pepper, scallions, and mint; use as a dipper instead of chips or crackers
EGGPLANT				
Slice off the ends, cut into ¾-inch slices, sprinkle evenly with salt, and lay in a colander to drain for 30 minutes; rinse to remove the salt, and dry; slice, chop, dice, mash, or puree	Chef's knife, colander	Cooked	Bake, roast, sauté, simmer, grill, stir-fry, braise, slow cooker	Mash into a dip; marinate and grill for a sandwich with tomatoes and smoked mozzarella; lightly bread and bake in a tomato sauce topped with parmesan; roast and stuff with a grain and pomegranate seed salad; simmer with tomatoes, onion, garlic, and balsamic vinegar, and puree into a soup
GARLIC				
Peel. Chop the cloves, thinly slice, mince, or smash and lightly salt to form a paste	Chef's knife	Raw/cooked	Roast, sauté, blanch, bake, stir-fry	Drizzle a head of garlic with olive oil, wrap in aluminum foil with a sprig of rosemary, and roast until soft and caramelized; sauté or roast chopped or thinly sliced garlic with vegetables, legumes, or grains; add to a soup with onions and thyme
GINGER				
Peel using a spoon and trim; slice, mince, or grate	Spoon, paring knife, fine grater or zester	Raw/cooked	Simmer, sauté, stir-fry	Add to broths and soups; grate finely to add to fruit with a squeeze of fresh lime juice; add to miso and garlic paste to rub on vegetables; gingerbread; add to sauces or jams

PREPPING OPTIONS	TOOLS	RAW/ COOKED	COOKING METHODS	SERVING IDEAS
GREEN BEANS				
Trim stem end; slice lengthwise or slice crosswise on the diagonal	Paring knife, chef's knife	Cooked	Blanch, sauté, simmer, bake, roast, stir-fry	Add to salads, soups, and grains; roast with olive oil, thyme, salt, pepper, and a squeeze of lemon juice
GREENS (SPINACH)				
Stack leaves, remove stems (not necessary for baby spinach), roll into a fat cigar shape, and thinly slice; gather slices together and mince	Chef's knife	Raw/cooked	Blanch, braise, sauté, simmer, stir-fry	Sauté in a little olive oil, salt, and pepper, then toss with cooked quinoa, yellow raisins, and a squeeze of lemon juice; add to soups, salads, sandwiches, and pasta
GREENS (SWISS CHARD, MUSTARD, DANDELION)				
Remove the central fibrous stem, if applicable, and stack several leaves on top of one another; fold in half lengthwise, roll into a fat cigar shape, and cut crosswise into wide or narrow ribbons; gather ribbons together and finely chop or mince	Chef's knife	Raw/cooked	Bake, blanch, braise, roast, sauté, simmer, steam	Use Swiss chard leaves like tortillas for rolling up grains and vegetables, cover with a pasta sauce and cheese, and bake; sauté Swiss chard stems separately with garlic, salt, and pepper, finished with a vinegar drizzle; sauté garlic and onion, add broth, salt, and pepper, then braise mustard greens until tender; sauté dandelion greens in olive oil, garlic, salt, pepper, and red pepper flakes
HERBS (BASIL, MINT, SAGE)				
Roll or stack to thinly slice; mince, chop	Chef's knife	Raw/cooked	Sauté, roast, simmer	Pesto; add to salads, vegetables, grains, legumes, pasta, and eggs; add to dressings and sauces; add to pizza and breads, such as flatbread
KALE				
Fold leaves over the central tough rib, and remove the rib using a knife (not necessary for baby kale); coarsely chop	Chef's knife	Raw/cooked	Sauté, blanch, bake, roast, stir-fry, simmer, braise, grill, steam	Pesto; baked kale chips; sauté with lemon, olives, and capers, and toss with quinoa; add to soup; braise with garlic, dried chipotle peppers, and tomatoes; add to a green smoothie
LEEKS				
Cut off and discard the top third part of the leek with tough, dark green leaves; halve lengthwise, and feather the layers under cold running water to remove dirt; slice into thin half-moons	Chef's knife	Raw/cooked	Sauté, roast	Raw in salads; add to sautéed or roasted vegetables; roast halves with olive oil, salt, and pepper

PREPPING OPTIONS	TOOLS	RAW/ COOKED	COOKING METHODS	SERVING IDEAS
MUSHROOMS (PORTOBELLO)				
Wipe clean with a paper towel; scrape out the gills using a spoon; leave whole or slice	Chef's knife, spoon	Raw/cooked	Grill, roast, sauté, braise, bake	Use in place of a bun for veggie burgers; stuff with vegetables, grains, or legumes; marinate in olive oil, balsamic vinegar, and garlic, then roast or grill
MUSHROOMS (SMALL)				
Wipe clean with a paper towel; slice, quarter, or mince	Chef's knife	Raw/cooked	Sauté, bake, stir-fry, roast, braise, grill	Coat with olive oil and a dusting of salt and pepper, and roast at 400°F until well browned; add to pasta and grain dishes; make mushroom risotto; stuff with peppers, garlic, bread crumbs, and parmesan cheese for an appetizer; use in casseroles
OLIVES (GREEN, NIÇOISE, KALAMATA)				
Slice, smash using the flat side of a chef's knife, coarsely chop, or leave whole	Chef's knife	Raw/cooked	Sauté, roast	Add to pastas, grains, vegetables, and legumes
ONION, SHALLOT				
Chop, dice, grate, or slice	Chef's knife	Raw/cooked	Bake, braise, fry, grill, roast, sauté, stir-fry, slow cooker	Stuff sweet onions with grains and other vegetables and roast; caramelize and add to sandwiches, burgers, grains, and legumes; make a flatbread with caramelized onions, goat cheese, and herbs
PEAS				
Pry the shells open using your nails or a small knife, and remove the peas; puree or leave whole	Food processor or blender	Raw/cooked	Bake, blanch, braise, sauté, simmer, steam, stir-fry	Add to pasta, casseroles, soup, and vegetable dishes; puree for a pea soup; lightly sauté with salt and pepper, and toss with mint; add to an asparagus quiche or omelet
PEAS (SUGAR SNAP, SNOW)				
Trim ends, and leave whole or thinly slice	Paring knife, chef's knife	Raw/cooked	Bake, braise, grill, roast, sauté, steam, stir-fry	Toss in olive oil, salt, and pepper, then grill and toss with chopped mint before serving; sauté, then sprinkle with sea salt; sauté in sesame oil, and finish with lemon, salt, pepper, and sesame seeds

PREPPING OPTIONS	TOOLS	RAW/COOKED	COOKING METHODS	SERVING IDEAS
PEPPERS (BELL)				
Place a pepper on a workspace with the stem facing up and cut off the side "lobes" and bottom; discard seeds, pith, and top (which should be all connected as one piece); cut into lengths; dice; puree	Chef's knife, food processor or blender	Raw/cooked	Roast, sauté, simmer, bake, grill, stir-fry, slow cooker	Roast and peel, halve, seed, and drizzle with olive oil, garlic, salt, and pepper; puree as soup; add to tomato sauces; stuff whole with grains and vegetables; add to salads, sandwiches, grains, legumes, and pasta; raw with a dip; add to bread; add to sauces such as aïoli
POTATOES (SWEET)				
Peel using a vegetable peeler; slice, dice, chop, grate, or puree	Chef's knife, vegetable peeler, food processor or blender, box grater	Cooked	Roast, bake, sauté, simmer, grill, steam, slow cooker	Baked and stuffed; puree for a sauce or soup or to add to pancake or muffin batter; add to stews and chili; enchiladas; tacos; roast, and add to warm salads; add to root vegetable roasts and gratins; baked sweet potato chips; sauté with butter and maple syrup; baked sweet potato fries; hash
POTATOES (WHITE, RED, YUKON GOLD, FINGERLING)				
Peel (or not), slice, dice, mash, puree, grate, or smash	Vegetable peeler, chef's knife, paring knife, potato masher, box grater, food processor (using pulse only)	Cooked	Bake, braise, fry, grill, roast, sauté, simmer, slow cooker, steam, stir-fry	Twice-baked potatoes whipped with soft cheese and topped with chives; cut into wedges, toss with olive oil, salt, and pepper, then roast until brown; grill potato slices to add to salads; smash roasted baby red potatoes, sprinkle with salt, pepper, and dried rosemary, then drizzle with olive oil; roast; hash browns
RADISHES				
Trim roots and tops; leave whole, halve, or thinly slice	Paring knife	Raw/cooked	Bake, braise, fry, stir-fry	Bake or roast with butter, salt, pepper, and parsley; add to salads
SCALLIONS				
Trim roots and remove any outer damaged sheath; leave whole, halve lengthwise, or chop	Paring knife, chef's knife	Raw/cooked	Braise, roast, grill, sauté, stir-fry	Toss in olive oil, salt, and pepper, then roast or grill; add to salads, soups, pasta, grains, pizza, or legume dishes; add to any kind of egg dish

PREPPING OPTIONS	TOOLS	RAW/ COOKED	COOKING METHODS	SERVING IDEAS
SQUASH (BUTTERNUT)				
Slice off ends, halve the squash crosswise just above the bulbous end, stand on end and peel using a sharp knife or vegetable peeler; scoop out seeds using a spoon; cut into wedges, chop, dice, puree	Chef's knife, food processor, blender, spoon, vegetable peeler	Cooked	Roas, sauté, steam, simmer, slow cooker	Stuff with grains and/or vegetables; add to salads, grains, legumes, and vegetables; soup; risotto
SQUASH (DELICATA)				
Slice off the ends, halve, and scrape out the seeds; slice into half-moons, or puree	Chef's knife, spoon, food processor or blender	Cooked	Roast, bake, sauté, simmer, grill, braise, steam, slow cooker, stir-fry	Soup; stuff scooped-out half with grains, dried fruits, and other vegetables; sprinkle with oil, garlic, salt, pepper, and cayenne, then roast; add to warm salads or bowls; use as a pizza topping; toss with pasta; add to tacos; puree to add to chilis and stews
SQUASH (SPAGHETTI)				
Halve and scoop out seeds and pulp with a spoon, or leave whole; after cooking, run the tines of a fork across the flesh to pull up "spaghetti" strands	Chef's knife, spoon, fork	Cooked	Roast, bake, slow cooker	Stuff with black beans, roasted red peppers, and onions, then top with cheese; toss strands with olive oil, parmesan cheese, salt, pepper, and roasted pumpkin seeds
SQUASH (ZUCCHINI, SUMMER)				
Trim the ends and chop, dice, or cut into rounds, wedges, or matchstick lengths; grate using the largest holes of a box grater; make long thin noodles using a vegetable peeler	Paring knife or chef's knife, box grater, food processor or blender, vegetable peeler	Raw/cooked	Bake, grill, roast, sauté, simmer, steam, stir-fry	Bake as fries: cut into wedges, then toss in olive oil, salt, pepper, oregano, and parmesan cheese; substitute thin slices for spaghetti, then toss with tomatoes, basil, and garlic; halve lengthwise, slightly hollow out to make boats, and stuff with vegetables and grains, topped with pasta sauce and cheese
TOMATOES				
To peel a tomato, using a paring knife, score the skin on the bottom of the tomato with an X, blanch in simmering water for 20 seconds, then dip in a bowl of ice water, peel starting at the X; slice, chop, dice, grate, or puree	Paring knife or chef's knife, box grater, food processor or blender	Raw/cooked	Bake, blanch, braise, fry, grill, roast, sauté, simmer, stir-fry	Stuff raw with chickpea or lentil salad; halve and slow-roast with garlic, salt, and pepper; salsa; caprese salad with fresh mozzarella, basil, and olive oil; bruschetta; gazpacho

WEIGHTS AND VOLUME CONVERSION TABLES

VOLUME EQUIVALENTS (LIQUID)

US Standard	US Standard (ounces)	Metric (approximate)
2 tablespoons	1 fl. oz.	30 mL
¼ cup	2 fl. oz.	60 mL
½ cup	4 fl. oz.	120 mL
1 cup	8 fl. oz.	240 mL
1½ cups	12 fl. oz.	355 mL
2 cups or 1 pint	16 fl. oz.	475 mL
4 cups or 1 quart	32 fl. oz.	1 L
1 gallon	128 fl. oz.	4 L

OVEN TEMPERATURES

Fahrenheit (F)	Celsius (C) (approximate)
250°F	120°C
300°F	150°C
325°F	165°C
350°F	180°C
375°F	190°C
400°F	200°C
425°F	220°C
450°F	230°C

VOLUME EQUIVALENTS (DRY)

US Standard	Metric (approximate)
⅛ teaspoon	0.5 mL
¼ teaspoon	1 mL
½ teaspoon	2 mL
¾ teaspoon	4 mL
1 teaspoon	5 mL
1 tablespoon	15 mL
¼ cup	59 mL
⅓ cup	79 mL
½ cup	118 mL
⅔ cup	156 mL
¾ cup	177 mL
1 cup	235 mL
2 cups or 1 pint	475 mL
3 cups	700 mL
4 cups or 1 quart	1 L

WEIGHT EQUIVALENTS

US Standard	Metric (approximate)
½ ounce	15 g
1 ounce	30 g
2 ounces	60 g
4 ounces	115 g
8 ounces	225 g
12 ounces	340 g
16 ounces or 1 pound	455 g

Index

About the Author

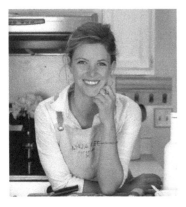

Chef Anja Lee Wittels is known for her passionate personality, particularly when it comes to anything food, wine, and coming together to eat and enjoy. Having loved cooking with Mom and Mimi (Grandma) at a young age, she quickly dove into working with a local caterer and one of Anja's biggest inspirations, Melanie. From then, whether catering with Melanie as a summer job, or cooking in restaurants and, quite often, for friends and family, Anja continued to expand her knowledge and passion for cooking. She also studied abroad in Lyon, France, where she spent a year sitting at the kitchen counter learning secret recipes from her Host Mom, Sylvie, and cooking in restaurants. Finally, she started her own catering and cooking class companies, and both businesses thrive in San Francisco and virtually all over the United States. She's cooked for the Golden State Warriors and the Cleveland Cavaliers and has even competed on the Food Network! Follow her and book cooking classes at AnjaLee.co.

Acknowledgments

Thank you to all of the brilliant souls in my life who helped make this happen. Special acknowledgments: to Manami, for helping me make this cookbook come to life; to Dina and team, for holding down the fort while I focused on this book; to Kelsey, for some *serious* recipe testing; to Liz and Scott, Mom, Breck and Kali, Mimi, and Spencer for being my other fantastic recipe testing guinea pigs; to Judith for being my backboard; and to my family, for always being a dream team support squad. I love you all dearly.

CPSIA information can be obtained
at www.ICGtesting.com
Printed in the USA
JSHW010211270521
15261JS00005B/32

9 781648 766625